PROSTATE CANCER

From Diagnosis to Treatment

Third Edition

ARTHUR CENTENO, M.D.

Addicus Books
Omaha, Nebraska

An Addicus Nonfiction Book

ISBN: 978-1-943886-84-5
Illustrations and typography by Jack Kusler

This book is not intended to be a substitute for a physician, nor do the authors intend to give advice contrary to that of an attending physician.

Library of Congress Cataloging-in-Publication Data

Names: Centeno, Arthur, 1953—author.
Title: Prostate cancer : from diagnosis to treatment / Arthur Centeno, M.D.
Description: Third edition. | Omaha, Nebraska : Addicus Books, [2018] | Includes bibliographical references and index.
Identifiers: LCCN 2018011563| ISBN 9781943886845 (alk. paper) | ISBN 9781943886975 (kindle) | ISBN 9781943886968 (epub)
Subjects: LCSH: Prostate—Cancer—Popular works.
Classification: LCC RC280.P7 C46 2018 |
DDC 616.99/463—dc23
LC record available at https://lccn.loc.gov/2018011563

Addicus Books, Inc.
P.O. Box 45327
Omaha, Nebraska 68145
www.AddicusBooks.com

Printed in the United States of America
10 9 8 7 6 5 4 3 2 1

To the memory of my late wife, Virginia, and to the memory of my patients who have lost their battles with cancer. They have taught me about the human spirit, the will to live, and the dignity of fighting the good fight.

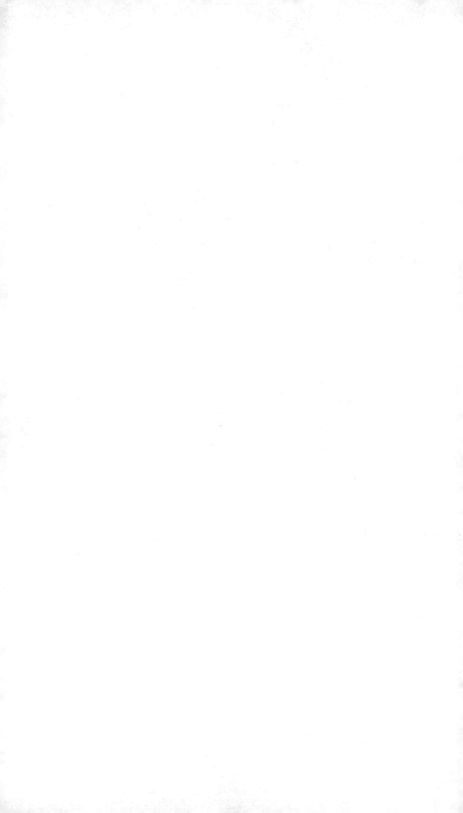

Contents

Introduction

If you have been diagnosed with prostate cancer, you are not alone. Some 165,000 men are diagnosed with the disease annually in the United States. A diagnosis of cancer is the beginning of a journey that none of us would choose to take. It is a journey that most of us begin with fear and trepidation. But, thanks to modern medicine, many of our fears can be put to rest. Much can be done to fight prostate cancer. And that fight is often won, especially when the cancer is diagnosed early.

Having treated thousands of patients, I have learned that one of the ways a patient can combat fear and anxiety is to become an active participant in his treatment. This means learning about the disease and the treatment options. The more you know, the less you face the unknown. Knowledge helps take away some of the fear.

It is my hope that this book will help you make smart decisions as you and your urologist move through treatment. Of course, no book can be a substitute for your doctor's expertise and advice. But with the information on these pages and in the scores of other excellent resources for prostate cancer patients and their loved ones, you can be an active partner in the disease's management and possibly in its cure.

What lies behind us and what lies ahead of us are tiny matters compared to what lies within us.

—Ralph Waldo Emerson
1803–1882

1   Prostate Cancer: An Overview

If you have been told that you have prostate cancer, your first reaction might well have been panic,
numbness, or despair. Many people experience a whirl
of emotions after receiving a cancer diagnosis. It's normal
to react this way. However, men who have had prostate
cancer will often talk positively about how their diagnosis
and recovery affected them emotionally.

Even though you might find this hard to believe
right now—there are thousands of prostate cancer survivors who will tell you that having had prostate cancer
eventually had a positive effect on them. They edu-
cated themselves about the disease and treatments, and
they discovered that knowledge is power. They learned
to use that power for their own health and well-being.
They forged new relationships and strengthened exist-
ing ones. They spoke to loved ones about their deep-
est feelings and greatest fears. They came to develop a
greater appreciation of life.

The Prostate Gland

To better understand prostate cancer, let's first examine the role of the prostate gland itself. The *prostate* is a
muscular gland about the size and shape of a walnut. It
is part of the urinary and reproductive systems and is located in the pelvis below the urinary bladder, just in front
of the rectum. The *urethra,* a tube that carries urine and

Prostate Gland

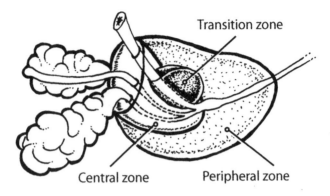

Transition zone

Central zone

Peripheral zone

semen out of the body through the penis, runs through the prostate.

Because the prostate is actually several small glands encased in the *prostate capsule,* it is sometimes described as having zones. Of these, the *peripheral zone,* or outer zone, is the largest and is where most prostate cancer begins. The *central zone* surrounds the ejaculatory ducts; less than 5 percent of prostate cancers originate here, but are usually more aggressive tumors. The *transition zone,* or innermost zone, surrounds the urethra; this is the area of the gland that grows as men age, often causing obstruction symptoms.

The Prostate and Urination

The health of the prostate can affect your ability to urinate. Because the prostate surrounds the urethra, prostate enlargement can squeeze the urethra, making urination difficult.

The urinary tract begins at the *kidneys,* the body's main filters. They cleanse impurities from about forty-five gallons of water every day. Most of this water is recirculated through the body, producing only about two quarts of waste in the form of urine.

Prostate Gland Side View

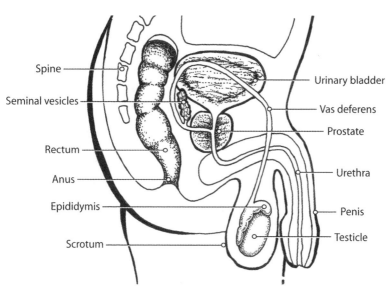

Urine travels to the *urinary bladder* through tubes called *ureters.* The bladder, located above the prostate, holds about a pint of urine. Urine empties into the urethra, which carries it through a muscle called the *urinary sphincter* and out through the penis. The urinary sphincter is responsible for continence, your ability to control the flow of urine.

The Prostate and Reproduction

Your prostate gland is small. About the size of an English walnut, it weighs between twenty and forty grams. By comparison, a first-class letter weighs about thirty grams. Small as it is, the prostate is essential for normal human reproduction. It adds important fluid and nutrients to sperm during ejaculation. To function properly, the prostate depends on male hormones, chiefly *testosterone.* This hormone is produced starting at puberty and is responsible for the traits usually associated with men such as body hair, deep voice, and muscles.

Prostate Gland Frontal View

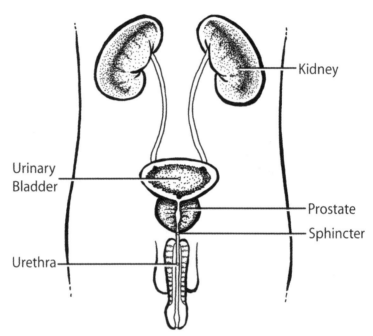

The prostate alone does not fuel the reproductive process. The *testicles* produce sperm and most of the testosterone upon which the prostate depends. Just before the male orgasm, muscles squeeze *seminal fluid* from the prostate and from the seminal vesicles. During ejaculation, sperm, carried by the seminal fluid, travel through the urethra and exit the penis.

Prostate Cancer

The general term *cancer* refers to a collection of cells that are growing out of control. Cancer cells grow past normal limits, and they don't die when they should. Instead, they divide and spread, sometimes uncontrollably. Such a growth is said to be *malignant*. These cancer cells can break away from a malignant tumor site and spread, or *metastasize,* to other organs. Cancer destroys normal tissue and creates new tumors as it spreads.

Preventing Prostate Cancer

Scientists have known that a high-fat, low-fiber diet greatly increases the likelihood of cancer. Research has shown that a healthful diet not only decreases the likelihood of cancer, it may slow cancer's growth. A southern Mediterranean diet that includes olive oil and cooked vegetables may prevent prostate and other cancers. The same is true for a Japanese diet—high in rice, fish, soy, vegetables, and green tea.

To reduce the risk of prostate cancer and other disorders, your daily diet should include at least five servings of fruits and vegetables from a variety of sources, minimal red meat, and no more than three servings of dairy products. Only 20 percent of your diet should come from fats.

Cancer spreads through the body's lymphatic system. *Lymph* is a fluid that bathes every living cell in the body. The lymphatic system fights cancer cells, killing and disposing of them. Sometimes, however, there are more cancer cells than the lymphatic system can handle, and the lymph vessels themselves become vehicles for spreading cancer.

Typically, prostate cancer starts in the outer zone of the prostate gland. Male hormones, especially testosterone, stimulate growth of both normal and cancerous cells in the prostate.

Stages of Prostate Cancer

When prostate cancer is diagnosed, the stage of the cancer is described as being *local, regional,* or *distant.* Local stage means the tumor is "localized" and there is no sign the cancer has spread outside the prostate. Regional stage refers to cancer that has spread from the prostate to nearby tissues. Distant stage refers to cancer that has spread to distant lymph nodes, bones, or other organs.

Survival Rates by Stage

- *Local stage:* about 4 out of 5 prostate cancers are found in this early stage. The 5-year survival rate for local stage prostate cancer is nearly 100 percent.

- *Regional stage:* the 5-year survival rate for regional stage prostate cancer is approximately 98 percent.
- *Distant stage:* the 5-year survival rate for distant stage prostate cancer is about 29 percent.

Most men with prostate cancer will live long, full lives. Many will never know they have it and will eventually die from unrelated causes.

Symptoms of Prostate Cancer

Early prostate cancer has no symptoms. You could be feeling quite well when you are diagnosed. For most men, the diagnosis comes as a complete surprise.

Malignant tumors in the prostate generally start out very small. It usually takes years for prostate cancers to grow large enough to obstruct the flow of urine. Fortunately, modern diagnostic methods can detect prostate cancer long before symptoms have a chance to develop.

Still, one or more of the following symptoms can indicate prostate cancer:

- Getting up at night to urinate
- Frequent urination during the day
- Weak or interrupted urinary flow
- Difficulty starting the urine stream
- Straining to urinate
- Feeling an urgent need to urinate
- Dribbling, leakage
- Pain or burning during urination
- Hematuria—blood in the urine
- Pain during ejaculation
- Less ejaculate (semen) than normal
- Impotence or less rigid erections

Although these symptoms do not always indicate prostate cancer, they should never be ignored. Prostate cancer that has spread beyond the gland itself can cause a range of symptoms, depending on where the cancer has spread. Symptoms may include pain that comes and goes in the back, ribs, hip, or shoulder.

Other symptoms include fatigue, weakness, and generalized aches and pains. Even though these symptoms are vague and could easily be harmless, don't ignore them. Too many men regard their symptoms as "normal signs of aging." It bears repeating: Do not ignore these symptoms. See your doctor right away if you have any of these symptoms.

Risk Factors for Prostate Cancer

Age

The greatest risk for prostate cancer is age. According to the American Cancer Society, prostate cancer is rare in men under age forty, but 60 percent of prostate cancers are found in men over sixty-five. The average age at the time of diagnosis is sixty-six. About 80 percent of men who reach age eighty have prostate cancer cells in their prostate glands, but that does not necessarily mean they will die of the disease.

Race and Ethnicity

In the United States, prostate cancer is more common in African-American men than in white men. White men have the second-highest rate of diagnoses, followed by Hispanic, American Indian/Alaska Native, and Asian/Pacific Islander men.

Family History

Up to 10 percent of prostate cancers can be linked to a man's family history. Having a father or brother diagnosed with prostate cancer, especially before age sixty, doubles a man's risk.

Occupation and Chemical Exposure

Though the evidence is inconclusive, it appears that employment in some occupations places men at higher risk for prostate cancer than the general population. These occupations include agricultural workers, firefighters, soap and perfume manufacturers, leather workers, mechanics, welders, and white-collar workers.

With the exception of white-collar workers, these occupations involve exposure to chemicals, including pesticides, herbicides, and fertilizers. Depending on the type, degree, and duration of exposure, toxins may damage cells to the point where they mutate and become cancerous. Exposure to the element cadmium, which interferes with zinc absorption, is also a potential risk. Men with prostate cancer tend to have lower levels of zinc in their bodies. For white-collar workers, the risk is linked to inactivity combined with unhealthy lifestyle choices.

Being Overweight

Currently, obesity is not considered a risk factor for prostate cancer; however, men who are obese tend to have more aggressive cancers when they are diagnosed. If you exercise regularly, keep it up; if you don't, ask your doctor to recommend an exercise plan. Exercise helps maintain hormone levels, prevents obesity, and enhances immune function. Men who exercise vigorously three times a week have a lower death rate from prostate cancer compared to men who do not exercise regularly.

Smoking

Studies do not show a definite link between smoking and prostate cancer; however, those who smoke and are diagnosed with prostate cancer often have more aggressive cancers. Former smokers may be at similar risk, depending on the length of time they smoked. Smoking can damage human cells. Health experts agree that stopping a tobacco habit is one of the best things you can do for your immediate and long-term well-being.

Prostate Cancer Statistics

Second to skin cancer, prostate cancer is the most commonly diagnosed cancer among men in the United States. According to the American Cancer Society, one out of nine men will be diagnosed with prostate cancer. Approximately 60 percent of cases are diagnosed in men aged 65 or older, and it is rare in men under age 40. The average age at diagnosis is 66.

Approximately 165,000 men in the United States are diagnosed annually. Compared to other types of cancer, prostate cancer grows slowly and offers a high potential for cure. One in forty-one will die of the disease.

2   Getting a Diagnosis

The cure rate for prostate cancer is high when the cancer is diagnosed early. Fortunately, men are being screened for the disease more than ever before. In the years before prostate cancer screening and early detection were available, up to one-third of the men who were diagnosed were found to have advanced prostate cancer. Today, advanced cancer is found in only about 5 percent of new cases. Simply put, screening and early detection are lifesavers.

Several diagnostic tests help your doctor determine whether you have prostate cancer. These tests typically start with a simple blood test and physical exam in a urologist's office. Then, if necessary, a urologist will conduct more-sophisticated tests to reach a diagnosis.

Digital Rectal Exam

One of the initial examinations a physician will perform is a *digital rectal exam (DRE)*. To perform this exam, a doctor will insert a gloved, lubricated index finger into the rectum, which is right behind the prostate gland. Using his finger, the doctor can feel the surface of the prostate gland; a normal prostate is soft, smooth, and symmetrical. The doctor will check for areas that may feel hard or uneven; he'll also be checking for lumps and enlargement of the gland.

These symptoms don't always indicate the presence of cancer. They may be an indication of other prostate

Digital Rectal Exam (DRE)

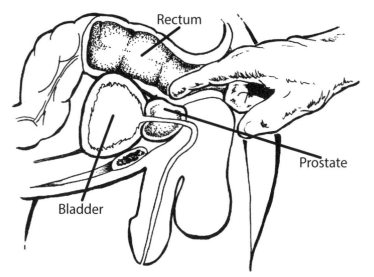

The normal prostate gland is soft and smooth. Most prostate cancers start in the outer "zone" of the prostate gland, and doctors are often able to feel lumps or other changes in the gland when performing a digital rectal exam (DRE).

disorders such as infection, stones, inflammation, or a noncancerous enlargement. In either case, additional tests will determine a diagnosis.

The location of abnormalities within the gland is important. Almost three-fourths of prostate cancers start in the gland's outer zone, which a doctor can feel. However, at least one-fourth of prostate cancers occur in an area of the prostate that a doctor cannot reach with a finger. That's why the PSA blood test is so important.

Prostate-Specific Antigen (PSA) Test

One of the most commonly used tests to determine the health of the prostate gland is a test that analyzes the level of *prostate-specific antigen (PSA)* in the bloodstream. An antigen is a substance that stimulates the body's immune response. These antigens are found in both normal and malignant tissue. Fluctuations of antigens sometimes indicate cancer.

All prostate cells, both normal and cancerous, produce PSA. However, cancerous cells multiply more quickly than normal cells; as a result, more PSA is produced. So an elevated PSA is a warning that something may be wrong and that more studies are needed. That "something" could be a number of things, including inflammation or infection; or it might be caused by recent activity that "massages" the prostate, such as riding a bicycle or motorcycle. Also, sexual intercourse can elevate your PSA by as much as 10 percent.

If your digital rectal exam is normal but your PSA is mildly elevated, your doctor will ask for a urine sample to see if you have a prostate infection *(prostatitis)*. If you do, the doctor will probably prescribe an antibiotic and do another PSA blood test several weeks after you've finished taking the antibiotics.

Some medical experts recommend a PSA blood test starting at age forty for African-American men and men with a family history of prostate cancer. Annual screenings for other men are recommended starting at age fifty.

What Is a Normal PSA Level?

A sensitive blood test is used to measure PSA levels. A "normal" PSA level is not the same for everyone (see guidelines on the following page). The level varies depending on age and ethnicity.

Not all the experts agree on these guidelines. Some say a level above 4.0 is suspicious regardless of the patient's age. Others advise men to have more tests if their first-time PSA is 2.5 or above.

Scientists have found several ways to interpret PSA test results to form a better idea of whether cancer is causing the PSA increase. One of these is called *PSA velocity (PSAV) test,* which compares PSA levels over time to see

PSA Screening Guidelines

Age	Normal PSA	African-American Normal PSA
40–50	2.5 or lower	2.0 or lower
50–60	3.5 or lower	3.0 or lower
60–70	4.5 or lower	4.0 or lower
70 and up	6.5 or lower	6.0 or lower

how quickly they are rising. Your doctor may suspect prostate cancer if your PSA rises.

Prostate Health Index

If your PSA test results are outside the normal range, your doctor may order a test called a *prostate health index (PHI)*. This simple blood test provides more accurate information than a standard PSA test, and it helps physicians determine whether a biopsy is needed.

If the PSA test or prostate health index test indicates you might have prostate cancer, you'll probably have at least two additional diagnostic procedures—a transrectal ultrasound (TRUS) and a needle biopsy.

Transrectal Ultrasound

For the *transrectal ultrasound (TRUS)* procedure, a doctor will insert a lubricated ultrasound probe into your rectum, which is just behind the prostate gland. Because ultrasound waves bounce off normal tissue differently than off malignant tissue, the TRUS probe creates a picture of the prostate and abnormalities it might contain. The doctor views the picture on a video screen.

The TRUS procedure shows the size of the prostate, but it can't see all types of tumors. Some prostate tumors are distinct lumps, which often show up on TRUS, but other prostate tumors are spread out, and TRUS seldom shows these. As a result, a normal TRUS could merely mean that you, like most men with prostate cancer, have lesions that are flat, small, and scattered.

For some men, the transrectal ultrasound is uncomfortable. If a man cannot tolerate the procedure easily, he may be given light anesthesia.

Needle Biopsy

A *needle biopsy* is a procedure that extracts tiny tissue samples with a needle. There are several types of biopsies. Most men tolerate biopsy procedures well, but if you know you have a low pain threshold, talk with your doctor about ways to relieve any discomfort during the biopsy. Don't feel timid about requesting one of the topical or local pain relievers available. If you wish to be given intravenous sedation to make you sleep during the procedure, your procedure will probably be performed in an outpatient surgery center.

Biopsy with Transrectal Ultrasound

This biopsy can find cancer that might be missed by a transrectal ultrasound alone. Therefore, many doctors do an ultrasound and a biopsy at the same time. The ultrasound images that are projected onto a video screen show them where to direct the biopsy needle, making the biopsy procedure more accurate.

The ultrasound device targets six different zones in the prostate, allowing the doctor to collect tissue samples from the entire gland. Suspicious areas, such as nodules, are targeted as well. The doctor uses a high-speed biopsy "gun," which is a long, thin, hollow, spring-loaded needle; it is inserted through the ultrasound probe, and the physician removes twelve to twenty-four small samples of suspicious tissue.

After these procedures, if doctors are still unsure whether cancer is present, they may repeat the TRUS and biopsy in the months ahead. Whether a urologist repeats these tests depends on several factors, including the doctor's level of suspicion about the presence of cancer, a man's age, his tolerance to biopsies, and the findings of previous biopsies.

After all diagnostic tests are performed, a *pathologist,* a physician who specializes in diagnosing diseases, examines biopsied tissues under a microscope. If cancer is present, the pathologist determines how aggressive it appears to be.

MRI Fusion Biopsy

Another biopsy technique, called an *MRI fusion biopsy,* incorporates an MRI (scan) image of the prostate with a real-time sonogram to target suspicious areas of the prostate. A sonogram uses ultrasound to view an internal organ.

Saturation Biopsy

If a needle biopsy does not result in the discovery of cancer, but your physician still suspects it, he or she may recommend a *saturation biopsy* in which twenty or more tissue samples are collected. For the saturation biopsy, the needle is inserted into the rectum and is guided by ultrasound technology. Watching on a video monitor, the physician can view the needle's path as it enters the prostate gland. Then, as each tissue sample is collected, it is labeled, according to which part of the gland it was taken from.

Research shows that prostate cancer is found in 40 percent of men who have saturation biopsies after having as many as three previous biopsies that showed no presence of cancer.

Percutaneous Needle Biopsy

In advance of surgery for prostate cancer, many doctors recommend a *percutaneous needle biopsy (PNB)* to sample lymph nodes and examine them to see whether cancer has spread. A percutaneous needle biopsy extracts tissue from deep pelvic lymph nodes. A long, thin needle is guided by a CT scan. If you have this procedure, you'll be given local anesthesia and probably intravenous sedation. Plan to take the day off. You'll probably be able to resume regular activities the next day.

Preparing for a Biopsy

Prior to the biopsy, your doctor will ask you for a list of medications you're currently taking—prescription and over-the-counter medications as well as supplements. For at least a week before your biopsy, avoid alcohol and don't take any medicines or supplements that can thin your blood and interfere with its ability to clot. These substances include drugs such as aspirin, ibuprofen (Motrin or Advil), and other nonsteroidal anti-inflammatory drugs (except Tylenol). Also avoid supplements containing vitamin E, fish oil, ginkgo biloba, or garlic. You'll also be instructed to temporarily discontinue blood thinners such as Coumadin.

To prevent infection, your doctor will prescribe antibiotics. In addition, you'll have a cleansing enema before the procedure.

After a Biopsy

Needle biopsies are usually outpatient procedures. You may receive a sedative, so arrange for someone to drive you home. There are few physical limitations after a biopsy. Your doctor will likely tell you that you can resume normal activity the next day. You'll continue to take antibiotics, so avoid alcohol during this time. The biopsy results should be available within two or three days.

Biopsy Risks, Complications, and Side Effects

Serious side effects from biopsies are rare. Some patients worry that a biopsy could cause the cancer to spread; however, there are no studies to date showing spread of disease from a needle biopsy. Severe bleeding or infection occurs less than 1 percent of the time. It's normal to find blood in your urine, semen, or stool for a few weeks after a prostate biopsy.

Rarely, an infection will move into the bloodstream and cause a high fever, shaking, and chills. This reaction, called *sepsis,* is a medical emergency, and can be fatal if not treated immediately. Another rare but serious biopsy complication is a urinary blockage. If this occurs, you will feel pain and be unable to pass urine. Seek medical help immediately if you experience either of these symptoms.

Diagnostic Scans

In addition to the diagnostic techniques just explained, your doctor may also have you undergo one or more scans that provide more specific information about your cancer; the purpose of this additional testing is to help your medical team recommend the best treatment.

Bone Scan

If your PSA is higher than 10, your doctor may want you to undergo a bone scan to determine whether cancer has spread to your bones. Some doctors recommend a bone scan for all prostate cancer patients with aggressive tumors.

To have this test, a radioactive substance is injected into a vein; the substance is absorbed by your body in areas of rapid bone growth. Cancer cells in the bone stimulate new bone growth. A special camera is used to look for "hot spots," bone that may show the presence of cancer. However, other conditions can show up as hot spots, including arthritis, healed bone fractures, and *Paget's disease,* a nonmalignant bone disorder in which bone cells grow out of control.

Computerized Tomography Scan (CT Scan)

A *computerized tomography scan (CT scan,* also called a *CAT scan)* is performed to assess the presence

17

of metastatic disease in the lymph nodes. For this test, a scanner moves around your body to take a series of high-tech X-rays. This scan provides detailed three-dimensional photos of tissues and organs inside the body with much greater accuracy than standard X-rays. The test is painless and noninvasive. It can be performed as an outpatient procedure.

Magnetic Resonance Imaging (MRI)

Like the CT scan, *magnetic resonance imaging (MRI)* produces a three-dimensional image, but uses magnetic waves rather than X-rays. Painless and noninvasive, an MRI can determine whether tissue abnormalities are cancerous or benign. An MRI can be performed as an outpatient procedure.

The MRI produces a loud, clanging sound as strong electromagnetic fields are switched off and on. Many patients wear earplugs or listen to music through headphones during the procedure. The test typically involves twenty to forty-five minutes of confinement in a tunnel-like structure. If you tend to be claustrophobic, you can ask your doctor to give you a light sedative. Some facilities have "open" MRI scanners, which aren't totally enclosed.

An *endorectal coil MRI* may be used to provide enhanced images. This MRI uses a latex (rubber) balloon with a central tube that contains wire coils. The device is inserted into the rectum; it then sends radio waves that provide high-quality images of the prostate and surrounding tissues. Most men find this exam no more uncomfortable than a digital rectal exam.

PET Scan

For *positron-emission tomography (PET) scans,* a sugar solution is injected into a vein and circulates through the blood. Because tumor cells use glucose as an energy source, the sugar solution gravitates to cancerous tissues. As a result, PET scans can locate tumors

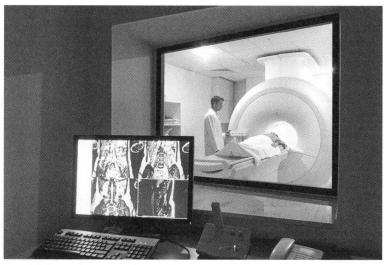

A magnetic resonance imaging (MRI) scan can detect cancer in the prostate gland and surrounding lymph nodes. The scan uses a large magnet, radio waves, and a computer to produce pictures; later, physicians view the scan results on a computer screen, as shown in the lower left corner.

and can tell how quickly they digest the sugar. The more rapid the digestion, the more likely it is that the cells are malignant.

However, PET scans are not used routinely in prostate cancer staging because prostate cancer cells are slow growing and less likely to show up on PET scans. This scan is usually not covered by health insurance.

Staging Prostate Cancer

The scans you undergo help your medical team determine the stage of your cancer. The stage is based on the cancer's size and the extent of its growth within or beyond the prostate. Knowing the stage helps doctors know how a cancer may progress and which type of treatment is best for you.

In the United States, there are two systems that doctors use to stage cancer. These staging systems, listed in the Appendix, are complex. You may want to ask your physician to help you understand the systems.

Grading Prostate Cancer

In the mid-1970s, Dr. Donald Gleason developed a grading system to measure the appearance and arrangement of prostate cancer cells viewed under a microscope. How the cells look can tell a pathologist a lot about how aggressive the cancer is likely to be.

Cell Makeup

Healthy cells are referred to as being *well differentiated.* This means a pathologist, using a microscope, can easily see the cell makeup—where one cell stops and another begins. Malignant cells are typically *poorly differentiated,* meaning their shapes and boundaries are not uniform and the normal cell structure is missing.

Assigning a Grade

To assign a grade to prostate cancer cells, the pathologist looks at the two largest areas of cancer in the tissue samples and assigns each of them a number from 1 to 5. Higher numbers are assigned to the more poorly differentiated (disorganized) cancer cells. The two numbers are then added to make up the *Gleason score.* The more disorganized the cells appear, the more aggressive the cancer and the higher the Gleason score.

Low Gleason scores of 2, 3, or 4 indicate relatively normal-appearing cell structures. Gleason scores of 5, 6, or 7 indicate moderately differentiated prostate cancer cells that are slower growing. Higher scores of 8, 9, or 10 indicate more-disorganized cells, which indicate a more aggressive and faster-growing cancer.

To discover whether your prostate cancer is confined to the prostate, your doctor will take into consideration such factors as your PSA, clinical stage, and Gleason score. With this information, doctors try to predict how your cancer might behave.

Choosing a Treatment Plan

The diagnosing procedures described in this chapter give your doctor important information about which treatment methods will be most effective for you. These treatments include hormone therapy, surgery, radiation therapy, and chemotherapy. Each of these treatments is discussed in later chapters. Treatment options are based on a man's age, general health, and stage of the cancer at the time of diagnosis.

Doctors Who Treat Prostate Cancer

During the course of your treatment for prostate cancer you may be treated by more than one physician. Doctors you may see include the following:

- *urologist,* who specializes in treatment of the urinary tract system and the male reproductive organs
- *radiation oncologist,* who treats cancer patients with radiation therapy
- *medical oncologist,* whose specialty is treating cancer with chemotherapy

Your urologist will continue routine appointments with you during the time you are being treated by a cancer specialist.

No Treatment Options

There are other options for older men who prefer to not undergo traditional treatment for prostate cancer. Instead, their doctors monitor their cancers and take action only if needed. Given that prostate cancers grow more slowly than other cancers, many men who have prostate cancer will not die from it.

Active Surveillance

Active surveillance actually involves no treatment, but rather careful monitoring of a man's prostate cancer. This is an option for men whose cancer is confined to the prostate, is slow growing, and is not causing symptoms.

To be more specific, a man under active surveillance will have a low-grade cancer with a Gleason score of 6 or lower. He should also have had a biopsy that shows three or fewer tissue samples that contain cancer. No single biopsy specimen should have more than 50 percent of its core tissue showing prostate cancer. The men in this category should also have PSAs of less than 10.

The follow-up monitoring of a low-grade cancer includes PSA tests every six months, a digital rectal exam every year, and a repeat prostate biopsy every one to three years; the need for a biopsy depends on a man's age and any progression in PSA test results.

Before going on active surveillance your physician may order a tissue-based genetic study to help decide on whether to treat the cancer. Genetic-based testing involves testing the makeup of tumor cells. This genetic test can predict the aggressiveness of a tumor and also predict future possibility of metastatic disease. With this additional information, you and your physician are better able to understand the risks of delaying treatment.

About 25 percent of men with prostate cancer are on active surveillance. Of those, some studies suggest that 33 percent will require treatment for prostate cancer within five years.

Watchful Waiting

Another approach to managing low-risk prostate cancer is *watchful waiting*. It involves monitoring prostate cancer that is not causing any symptoms or problems. Treatment begins only if symptoms occur. Many men on watchful waiting are elderly and will not require treatment.

3   Hormone Therapy

Hormone therapy is an effective tool in treating prostate cancer. Because hormone therapy acts to stabilize cancer growth, it is often given before primary treatments such as surgery or radiation. Hormone therapy enhances the effectiveness of both surgery and radiation. Hormone treatment may also be given after surgery or radiation so it can continue to block the hormones that feed cancer cells. In some cases, hormone therapy may be given alone.

How Hormone Therapy Works

Hormone therapy shrinks tumors and the prostate gland itself by blocking the production of male hormones, called *androgens.* The prostate gland needs these hormones to function, and cancer cells need these hormones to survive. Even when cancer cells have spread outside the prostate gland, they cannot reproduce without male hormones to "feed" them. As cancer cells die, they are not replaced if they are deprived of androgens.

Why then is hormone therapy not a cure-all for prostate cancer? Unfortunately, as some cancer cells grow, they mutate—changing in such a way that they no longer need male hormones to grow. These cells "learn" to survive and thrive without hormones. These cancer cells are called *androgen independent* because they can survive without male hormones. It's not known why some men develop only a small number of androgen-independent cells while other men develop many.

Hormone Therapy

Hormone therapy suppresses the production of male hormones, known as *androgens*. The androgen with which you are likely most familiar is testosterone. Nearly 95 percent of androgens are produced by the testicles; about 5 percent are produced by the adrenal glands and by other sites in the body.

When Is Hormone Therapy Given?

Hormone therapy is given when a man has an intermediate to high risk of cancer recurrence. Risk factors include a man's PSA level, his Gleason score, and the extent of any spreading of the cancer outside the prostate gland, including into nearby lymph nodes. The Gleason score refers to the grade of a cancer; low-grade cancers tend to grow slowly. High-grade cancers are more aggressive and grow faster.

It is common to receive hormone therapy prior to and after surgery. Some men may receive hormone therapy before, during, and after radiation treatments. Hormone therapy may be used alone in men who have had a cancer recurrence after surgery or radiation. It may also be used alone in men who may not be candidates for surgery or radiation.

The length of time a man receives hormone therapy depends on his overall health and the extent of his cancer. Treatments are given by injection. Some men may receive a shot monthly; others may receive a shot every few months. In some cases, men may stay on hormone therapy for years, or possibly for the rest of their lives.

Intermittent Hormone Therapy

Some men are given *intermittent hormone therapy*— treatments that are given in cycles, rather than continuously. This intermittent therapy gives men a break from side effects of hormone therapy. The timing of treatment cycles depends on a man's overall health and the extent of his cancer. Some patients do well enough after a year of hormone therapy to stop treatments for years before resuming them.

Secondary Hormone Treatments

If hormone therapy stops working, other drugs, called *secondary hormone manipulators,* can be used to treat advanced prostate cancer. These drugs work to manipulate testosterone differently from previous rounds of hormone therapy. The drugs are given in pill form.

Side Effects of Hormone Therapy

When you undergo hormone therapy for prostate cancer, your body will respond to the drop in your level of male hormones. Most of these side effects disappear or lessen after you stop hormone therapy. The following are symptoms you may experience:

- fatigue
- weakness
- confusion
- trouble concentrating
- mood swings
- hot flashes and sweating
- impotence and loss of sex drive
- shrinkage of the testicles and penis
- loss of muscle mass
- breast tenderness or enlargement
- weight gain

Of these symptoms, hot flashes and loss of sex drive are the most common. Another side effect is loss of bone mass. Both cancer and its treatment can cause bone loss, increasing the risk of breaking bones. Your physician may talk to you about medications for such side effects.

Note: if you undergo hormone therapy to reduce testosterone production, your voice will not get higher. Nor will hormone therapy regrow hair you may have lost in the past.

Removal of Testicles

Another way to stop production of male hormones is surgical removal of the testicles. Called an *orchiectomy,* this surgical procedure is rarely performed nowadays, but it may be an option for some men who want to avoid a continuing treatment such as hormone therapy. After the removal of testicles, a man's testosterone levels drop dramatically in three to twelve hours.

The procedure is commonly performed on an outpatient basis. Complications are rare and recovery is usually rapid.

Are You a Candidate for Hormone Therapy?

Hormone therapy may be recommended if your PSA level is 10 or higher or if your Gleason score is 6 or higher; both of these factors place you at moderate to high risk for a cancer recurrence. You may benefit from hormone therapy if:

- You want more time to consider treatment options.
- Your physician wishes to decrease tumor size before prostate gland removal or radiation therapy.
- You wish to avoid invasive treatments such as surgery or internal radiation.
- Your PSA rises significantly after surgery or radiation. (Such an increase does not always mean cancer has recurred.)

In summary, hormone therapy is used to control prostate cancer by stopping or slowing the growth of prostate cancer cells. Hormone therapy is often effective in combination with other primary treatments such as surgery and radiation therapy.

4 Surgery for Prostate Cancer

Perhaps, in consultation with your surgeon, you have chosen surgery for treating your prostate cancer. Among men with early-stage prostate cancer, surgery to remove the prostate gland is the most commonly chosen treatment.

This surgery is called a *radical prostatectomy*. In medicine, the term *radical* refers to the removal of the source of a disease; *prostatectomy* is the medical term for removal of the prostate gland. In this operation, the surgeon removes the entire prostate gland along with some tissues around it, including lymph nodes and seminal vesicles—the small glands containing fluid that is part of semen. There are several surgical approaches for removing the prostate gland. Each approach to the operation typically takes two to three hours, and the hospital stay is usually overnight.

Radical Robotic Prostatectomy

In the United States, radical robotic prostatectomy has become the most-performed surgery for prostate gland removal. A surgeon uses robotic arms to perform the operation. Several small incisions are made in the abdomen, then the surgeons uses robotic arms to remove the entire prostate gland as well as some surrounding tissues.

During the robotic surgery, the surgeon is guided by a small camera so that he or she can see the prostate and

Robotic Surgery Incision

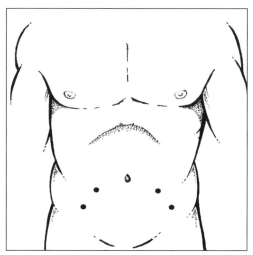

For robotic surgery, robotic arms reach the prostate gland through tiny incisions in the abdomen. This operation is less invasive and results in quicker recovery.

surrounding tissues on a video monitor. The advantages of robotic surgery include:

- less pain
- less blood loss
- improved visibility for the surgeon during the procedure
- smaller incisions
- faster recovery—a patient usually goes home the next day

There are disadvantages as well:

- Surgeons can't actually feel the tissue.
- Special equipment is needed.
- Tools inserted through the tube have a limited range of motion.
- Surgeons need special training for using the robotic equipment.

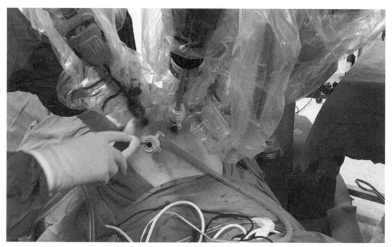

Robotic surgery is the most commonly used approach for removal of the prostate gland. Healing is faster compared to an operation with a large incision.

Sparing Nerves

In any operation to remove the prostate gland, a surgeon will try to preserve the *nerve bundles* on each side of the prostate gland. These nerves control a man's ability to have an erection. In years past, these nerves were almost always cut during a radical prostatectomy, and patients had to live with permanent impotence.

Now, with robotic surgery, surgeons can operate with precision, often preserving both nerve bundles or at least one of them. When a cancer appears to be located on only one side of the prostate, a surgeon may be able to leave the nerves intact on the opposite side.

Robotics Training and Equipment

The robotic approach requires that a medical center have the specialized robotic equipment and surgeons who are skilled in performing robotic surgery. Fortunately, most major medical centers employ experienced robotic prostatectomy surgeons and have the needed equipment.

Open Surgery Incision

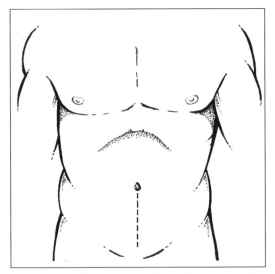

An open surgery to remove the prostate, performed through an eight- to ten-inch incision in the lower abdomen.

Laparoscopic Prostatectomy

The *laparoscopic* approach does not use a robot; however, a surgeon makes only small incisions across the abdomen. Then, by inserting a tiny camera that allows the surgeon to watch a video monitor for guidance while using surgical instruments.

Open Prostatectomy

The procedure known as an *open prostatectomy* was more commonly performed before the development of robotic surgery. This procedure is a major operation, in which a surgeon removes the prostate through an eight- to ten-inch incision, made from the navel down to the pubic bone. During the open operation, the prostate, seminal vesicles, and pelvic lymph nodes are removed. This open surgery requires a longer recovery period, usually several weeks, compared to the less-invasive approaches.

Cryosurgery

Cryosurgery, also known as *cryoablation*—"destruction by freezing"—is perhaps best known for its role in skin cancer treatment. Cryoablation has been used since the 1960s to remove skin tumors and precancerous moles. The same principle is at work when cryoablation is used to destroy internal cancers such as those of the prostate. In these procedures, doctors kill the cancer cells by applying super-cooled instruments directly into the prostate gland. Cryosurgery is typically performed on an outpatient basis.

In 2002, the American Urological Association deemed cryoablation of the prostate a "standard" rather than "investigational" procedure. However, today, the treatment is rarely used as a primary way to treat prostate cancer. Among other problems, cryosurgery has resulted in an impotency rate that exceeds 90 percent.

Are You a Candidate for Surgery?

You're most likely to benefit from surgery to remove the prostate if:

- your cancer is confined to the prostate gland
- you have fairly low-grade disease (Gleason score of 6 or less)
- your PSA level is 4 or less
- you're in your early seventies or younger
- you're in good overall health with a life expectancy of at least fifteen more years

There are exceptions to these guidelines. You may still be a candidate for surgery if the cancer has spread to the seminal vessels or you have a higher PSA level and a higher Gleason score.

If you believe you might be a candidate for surgery and your doctor doesn't agree, find out why. If you're not satisfied with the answer, get a second opinion. Do your own research and talk to prostate cancer survivors.

Preparation for Your Surgery

Your preparation for any of the types of surgeries will be similar. Your doctor will usually schedule surgery approximately two months after a needle biopsy. Prior to your operation, your doctor will provide instructions for you to follow

Hormone Therapy

As mentioned in the previous chapter, before surgery, you may undergo hormonal therapy to shrink the prostate gland along with cancerous tumors. Hormone treatment may improve the outcome of surgery, especially in cases in which aggressive tumors have spread locally.

Taking Routine Medications

Your surgeon's office will advise you on whether to take regular medications in the days before the surgery. For example, if you take a blood-thinning medication, your doctor may advise you to stop taking it prior to your surgery because blood thinners promote bleeding.

Preventing Blood Clots

Be sure to let your doctor know if you have ever had blood clots. This information helps the anesthesiologist and the surgeon take extra precautions during surgery. To further reduce the risk of blood clots, your doctor may have you wear *pneumatic stockings* during surgery and for a few days after. These stockings improve blood circulation by repeatedly inflating and deflating.

Other Preparations

To guard against infection, you'll take antibiotics before and after your operation. Your doctor may ask you to have an enema or take a laxative, or both, the night before surgery. You will be asked to not eat for at least twelve hours before the operation. You might also be given a special antiseptic soap for showering before surgery.

Undergoing Surgery

Soon after your arrival at the hospital, you will change into a hospital gown and the medical staff will make preparations for your operation. An intravenous (IV) line will be inserted into a vein in your arm. Medications, including your anesthesia, will be delivered through this IV.

You may receive general anesthetic through the IV line, or you may receive what's called *epidural anesthesia* that numbs the lower part of your body. To receive this anesthesia, a small area on your back will first be numbed with a local anesthetic. Then, a needle is inserted into the area surrounding the spinal cord in the lower back. A small tube is threaded through the needle into the epidural space at the base of your spine. The epidural space contains nerves running from your spine to your lower body. Epidural anesthesia prolongs recovery of bowel functions and sometimes requires an additional day or two in the hospital.

As mentioned earlier, during surgery, a surgeon removes not only the prostate gland but also surrounding tissues that include seminal vesicles and, in some cases, lymph nodes. Each of the types of surgery to remove the prostate gland takes two to three hours.

During the surgery, part of the urethra will be removed. The urethra is the duct that carries urine and is surrounded by the prostate. The surgeon will suture the remaining urethra to the bladder neck; this new connection is called an *anastomosis* and you'll need to protect it well during healing in the weeks ahead.

The surgeon will insert a Foley catheter through the penis into the bladder. While the catheter is in place, urine will bypass the anastomosis so it can heal properly.

After Your Operation

After your operation you'll spend an hour or more in the recovery room, where your vital signs will be monitored until the general anesthetic wears off. You'll still have an IV in your arm for receiving fluids and medication.

You'll wake up to find several other tubes have been inserted. One or two of them will be drains placed during surgery to suction fluids that may have built up in the abdomen. These drains are usually removed before you leave the hospital. In some cases, you may leave the hospital with a drain.

It is rare to have an allergic reaction to an anesthetic used during surgery, but it may occur. Allergic symptoms range from fever or a rash to swelling of the tongue and lips. If you notice any of these symptoms after you awake from the surgery, be sure to tell a nurse.

Managing Pain

Pain management begins in the hospital immediately after your surgery. Adequate pain control is important. Enduring severe pain can actually interfere with healing and put you at risk for complications. Pain limits your ability to breathe deeply, cough, and move around—all necessary for normal healing. If you had an epidural anesthesia, the epidural tube may remain in place for pain relief.

Another form of pain management, a *patient-controlled analgesia (PCA) pump* allows you to control the delivery of your pain medication. When you press a button, the pump delivers pain medication, often morphine. The device has built-in safeguards, so you cannot use it too much.

If you must rely on hospital staff to administer pain medication, don't be timid. You've just had major surgery on your midsection, and you need not be in pain. Before surgery, discuss your concerns about pain and medication with your surgeon. Don't wait until after your surgery, when you're groggy.

If you are prescribed pain medication to take at home, use it. There is no need for you to suffer through the pain. The best advice is: don't wait for pain to become intense before taking pain medication. Try to stay ahead of the pain.

As mentioned earlier, there is less pain with robotic surgery; the incision is smaller and the incision site is injected with long-acting local anesthetic agents. The less pain you have, the less pain medication you'll need.

Preventing Deep Venous Thrombosis

After your surgery, hospital staff will work with you to prevent blood clots in the deep veins of your legs— these clots are called *deep venous thrombosis (DVT)*. With the guidance of nurses, you'll be asked to get out of bed and move about because mobility keeps your blood circulating, avoiding the formation of clots. Not only are blood clots painful, they can be deadly if a clot breaks off and travels to your heart or to a lung. You'll be encouraged to walk for a few minutes every hour as soon as you're alert after surgery and for the entire time you're in the hospital.

Side Effects of Prostate Surgery

It's normal to have side effects after surgery. Not everyone experiences side effects in the same way; side effects vary among people. Potential side effects from prostate surgery include the following:

Incontinence

After surgery to remove the prostate gland, approximately 70 percent of men will have some degree of *stress incontinence*—urine loss caused by coughing, sneezing, or lifting. This condition usually resolves over a period of weeks to months following surgery.

See chapter 7 for more details about coping with incontinence.

Impotence

Most men experience impotence—erectile dysfunction—after prostate surgery. Being impotent after surgery does *not* mean that your sex life is over. Sex can still be pleasurable. Impotence refers only to the ability to have an erection, but it does not affect physical sensation, arousal, or the ability to have an orgasm.

The risk of impotence is about 30 percent for men in their forties, and it rises with age to about 80 percent for men in their seventies. If both nerve bundles near the prostate are spared during surgery, 75 percent of men can expect to return to their previous sexual function. If one bundle is preserved, 50 percent can expect to return to their ability to get an erection prior to surgery.

For details on coping with impotence, see chapter 7.

Change in Orgasm

After the prostate gland has been removed, a man does not have an ejaculatory emission. He will still feel the sensation of orgasm; however, there is no ejaculation of semen. Some men do find that orgasms become less intense and may "fade" with time.

Loss of Fertility

After prostate surgery, the body still produces sperm in the testicles, but it has no way to ejaculate because the tubes that carry semen have been severed. Therefore fathering a child in the conventional way is not possible. This is usually not a problem for older men; however, younger men might wish to talk to their doctors about storing sperm in a sperm bank prior to surgery.

Lymphedema

This side effect is rare but possible. *Lymphedema* (swelling) can result from any surgery in which lymph nodes were removed. After these nodes are removed in prostate surgery, fluid may build up in the legs or genital area. This may cause discomfort. Lymphedema can often be treated with physical therapy, but may never go away completely.

Slight Change in Penis Length

The penis *may* be slightly shorter after prostate cancer surgery. This is because part of the urethra is removed during surgery; however, most men do not see a difference in penis length after surgery.

Potential Complications

The potential risk for complications after surgery are greater than for after other forms of treatment for prostate cancer. The following complications are not common, but may occur.

- *Urethral stricture.* A stricture is a narrowing of the urethra caused by scar tissue that forms after surgery. The risk is lower than 10 percent, and the urethra can be "dilated" by a urologist in an outpatient procedure.

- *Deep venous thrombosis (DVT)*—Blood clots develop in the deep veins of the legs. Risk is about 10 percent, much lower when blood-thinning medication is used along with pneumatic stockings. These stockings use cuffs around the legs that fill with air and squeeze your legs. This increases blood flow through the legs and helps prevent blood clots.

- *Reaction to epidural anesthesia.* This is rare, but breathing difficulty and infection can occur.

- *Bowel injury.* The risk is about one-half of 1 percent. Such injury can likely be repaired during your operation.

Other rare complications include urinary tract infections, stomach ulcers, pneumonia, and allergic reactions to medication. The risk of death is less than one-half of 1 percent. The risk of other life-threatening complications is lower than 1 percent.

When to Seek Medical Attention

After your operation, seek medical attention immediately if you have:

- nausea
- vomiting
- difficulty breathing
- fever over 100 degrees
- chills
- rash—anywhere on the body (usually an allergic response to medications)
- any swelling or redness at the incision sites
- shortness of breath
- pain or swelling in one or both legs

If you have any of these symptoms in the middle of the night, don't wait until morning to seek medical attention. Go to an emergency room. Also, you should get medical attention if you cough up blood. This could indicate blood clots, which can be fatal. Often, blood clots can be treated with anticoagulant (anticlotting) medication that is usually effective when started immediately.

Also, seek medical attention if your catheter is blocked. This is a medical emergency. The catheter will need to be irrigated by medical professionals. Never attempt to remove a catheter yourself.

At Home after Surgery

Typically, after surgery, you will stay overnight in the hospital and go home the next day. You'll be given instructions—guidelines for diet, exercise, and bathing. Following are some general guidelines you'll be asked to follow during your recovery.

Preventing Blood Clots

After you're at home, you'll still need to continue the regimen to avoid blood clots. Frequent short walks will go a long way toward preventing blood clots. Also, avoid sitting for too long on a firm surface with your legs hanging over the edge; this can restrict blood circulation in your legs. Elevate your legs as much as possible.

Caring for a Foley Catheter

You'll leave the hospital with the Foley catheter still in place. It will remain in place for seven to ten days after your surgery. Although catheters can be uncomfortable, most men tolerate them well.

The catheter does require care. Your doctor will give you detailed instructions to follow at home until the catheter is removed. The catheter has two bags to collect urine—a larger bag to use at night and a smaller bag for daytime drainage. A tube connects the catheter to whichever drainage bag is in use. Follow these instructions:

- Never attempt to adjust or remove the catheter yourself. If the catheter is pulled loose or removed too soon, permanent incontinence—which is otherwise quite rare—could result.

- While the catheter is in place, take showers rather than tub baths and don't get into a swimming pool, Jacuzzi, or sauna.

- Empty the drainage bags often to keep urine from backing up into your bladder. Drain the smaller bag every three to four hours; drain the larger bag every eight hours.

- Don't pull on the catheter, and be sure there's enough slack in the tube so that you won't pull it out accidentally in your sleep.

During the second week after surgery, your bladder may start to "rebel" against the catheter. You may experience bladder spasms—uncomfortable cramping in

Foley Catheter

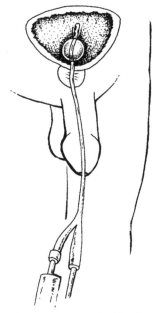

A Foley catheter is used to drain urine from the bladder when normal urination is disrupted. The catheter is threaded through the urethra and into the bladder.

the muscles that surround the urethra. The pain is felt in the lower abdomen and it may come and go; some men experience burning sensations. These spasms should resolve after your catheter is removed. Meanwhile, take the medications you've been prescribed, drink fluids as prescribed, and take four to six short walks each day without exhausting yourself. This light exercise keeps your blood moving.

After your catheter is removed, you'll notice some incontinence—the loss of bladder control that causes urine leakage. Even though this leakage is often temporary, it is an inconvenience and can be embarrassing.

Details on managing incontinence are given in chapter 7.

Preventing Infection

Most healing of your incision occurs within six weeks after surgery, but it will continue to heal for up to a year. Infections at the incision site are uncommon, but if your incision becomes tender or puffy, tell your health care provider right away. Antibiotic medication will usually take care of the problem.

Keeping Bowels Regular

After surgery, the part of the rectum next to the prostate gland will be fragile as it heals. It may be a few days after surgery before you have a bowel movement, which should be painless if you take stool softeners, according to your doctor's instructions. Avoid straining, which could injure the rectum.

Try to have a bowel movement every day. Use a stool softener if needed. Use laxatives only as directed by your doctor. Drinking adequate fluids and getting the right amount of dietary fiber can keep you from becoming constipated. For three months after your operation, do not have an enema or take your temperature rectally.

Resuming Daily Activities

Take it easy during the first week. This may be a good time to catch up on television programs or reading materials. You can probably return to your normal diet as long as it doesn't make you constipated. Generally, surgeons will recommend that you avoid driving for one week or while the Foley catheter is in place.

In the second week, when you'll likely feel better, you may be inclined to be more active. Still, doctors recommend staying off your feet as much as possible and doing nothing more strenuous than frequent short walks throughout the day.

Within two to four weeks after going home, you should be able to return to most of your usual routine, unless it is strenuous. You should be able to return to work after two to four weeks if you have a desk job; your doctor may instruct you to stay home a few weeks longer if your job requires heavy lifting or being on your feet a lot. Don't lift anything over ten pounds for the first six weeks.

Wait at least six weeks to play golf or tennis, bowl, lift weights, or ride a bicycle. Other physical activities can be resumed on the advice of your surgeon.

Follow-Up Doctor Visits

You'll likely see your urologist a week to ten days after surgery. At this time, he or she will examine your incision and remove your sutures. Your Foley catheter may also be removed. When the catheter is first removed, you will likely have temporary stress incontinence—urine leakage; this leakage may occur when you sneeze or when you stand up after sitting.

During a follow-up visit, you will receive details of your pathology report. This lab report provides details on the nature and extent of your cancer. As often as every three months for the first year, you'll have follow-up visits with your doctor. Then, you will likely have follow-up visits yearly.

Tests during Follow-Up Visits

During your postsurgical visits your doctor will likely perform a digital rectal exam (DRE) and a PSA blood test. The doctor will be checking for any evidence of complications from your treatment and will also check for any possible cancer recurrence. Your doctor will ask you about any urinary symptoms such as frequent urination, slow stream, leakage of urine, and burning sensations when urinating. You'll also likely be asked about any bowel symptoms such as diarrhea and blood or mucus in your stool.

5 Radiation Therapy

L ike surgery, radiation therapy is an effective treatment for prostate cancer. If you're a good candidate for radiation therapy, you and your urologist may choose it over surgery.

As part of radiation therapy, cancerous tissue is targeted with sophisticated computers and scanning devices. This makes it possible for radiation oncologists to focus on destroying cancer cells while minimizing damage to healthy tissues.

The two basic types of radiation treatment are *internal treatment* and *external treatment*. The internal treatment is called *brachytherapy*. The external type is called *external beam radiation therapy (EBRT or IMRT)*.

Internal Radiation Treatment

Internal radiation, called *brachytherapy,* involves the placement of tiny radioactive seeds directly into the prostate gland. The seeds deliver radiation for up to ten months. Because the seeds lose their radioactivity, there is no need to remove them.

Brachytherapy allows a physician to use a high dose of radiation to treat a smaller area in a one-time procedure, compared to external beam therapy, which is typically given over seven to eight weeks.

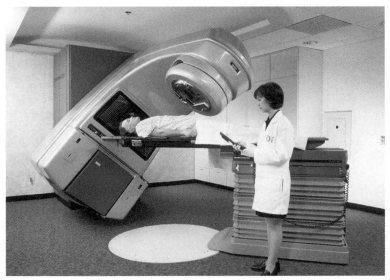

This photo represents a man undergoing external beam radiation therapy.
Photo courtesy of Varian Medical Systems of Palo Alto, California

Preparing for Brachytherapy

Prior to the brachytherapy procedure, you will have a *planning study*. To begin, a physician inserts an ultrasound probe into your rectum. The probe projects images onto a video monitor. Using computer software, the doctor determines where to place the radioactive seeds. The radiation dosage for the seeds is also calculated.

Preparing for brachytherapy is similar to preparing for prostate surgery. Usually, you'll wait eight to twelve weeks after you have begun hormone therapy before having brachytherapy. This gives the hormone treatment time to shrink the prostate.

You'll also start taking antibiotics prior to treatments to prevent infection. You'll be instructed when to stop taking drugs or supplements that might interfere with your treatment. Some doctors tell their radiation therapy patients to stop taking antioxidant supplements (vitamins C, E, and selenium), which may interfere with cancer-cell destruction.

Undergoing Brachytherapy

After you have received anesthesia, the urologist begins the procedure to insert the radioactive seeds into your prostate gland. First, an ultrasound probe is inserted in the rectum; this allows the urologist to see the prostate gland on a video monitor. A template grid is attached to the probe and fitted to the perineum, the area between the scrotum and rectum. The grids consist of rows and columns of tiny holes that provide a guide for the urologist to insert needles, pre-loaded with radioactive seeds. After the seeds inserted into the prostate gland, the needles are withdrawn. Depending on the size of the gland, 70 to 120 seeds are implanted.

The procedure to insert the radioactive seeds takes about two hours. The seeds stay in place permanently. They will deliver radiation to the prostate for up to ten months.

After Brachytherapy

After your brachytherapy procedure, you'll spend an hour or more in the recovery room until the general anesthetic wears off. You'll be given pain medication, and you'll probably receive oral antibiotics to take for several days. You'll likely go home the day of your procedure or the next day. Your surgeon will give you instructions to follow at home; you may be able to resume most of your routine activities in three to four days.

Some men who have had seed implants are concerned that they might be "radioactive." However, it's unlikely that radiation could harm others you come into contact with. Still, to be on the safe side, avoid close contact with babies, small children, and pregnant women for several months after treatment. To avoid any possible danger to children, some men wear lead-lined underwear for three months following their procedure.

Your doctor will likely give you guidelines for resuming sexual activity. Typically, you'll be asked to wait

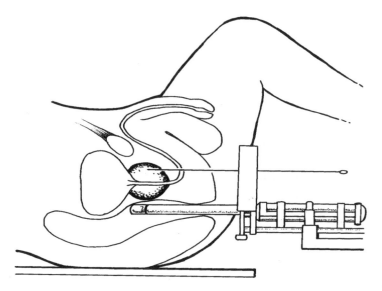

During a seed implant, an ultrasound probe, inserted in the rectum, helps the physician guide needle-like instruments in the prostate, where the radioactive seeds are delivered.

four to six weeks before having sex; condoms are recommended for four to six months following the procedure.

Follow-Up after Brachytherapy

After brachytherapy, you'll need to see your radiation oncologist every three to six months for a digital rectal exam and a PSA blood test. Your oncologist will watch for any complications from treatment and for possible recurrence of cancer.

Your oncologist will probably do a CT scan a month after treatment. He or she will check for any "cold spots," areas that the seeds are not reaching with radiation. If a cold spot is discovered, your oncologist may wish to monitor the cold spot or supplement the seed implant with external beam radiation.

> ## Hormonal Treatment Prior to Radiation
>
> Prostate cancer patients will often undergo *hormonal therapy* for several months before radiation begins. Hormonal therapy shrinks prostate tissues by depriving them of male hormones. By shrinking the gland, the area to receive radiation will be smaller. This means less radiation is needed and healthy tissues are less likely to be damaged.
>
> Doctors believe the hormone therapy also increases the kill rate of cancer cells when radiation is given. In short, hormone treatment makes radiation therapy more effective.

External Beam Radiation Therapy

The other basic type of radiation therapy is *external beam radiation therapy,* also called *EBRT* or *IMRT.* This painless form of treatment aims radiation beams at the prostate gland from outside the body. Treatments typically are given five days a week, Monday through Friday, over a seven- to eight-week period. For well-chosen radiation candidates, EBRT is as effective and safe as seed implantation. That's because newer techniques to deliver radiation allow for much greater precision than in years past. This means less chance of damaging tissues of the rectum, bladder, urethra, and other structures.

The most commonly used form of external beam radiation is called *intensity-modulated radiation therapy (IMRT).* As with internal radiation, this form of treatment also uses scanning and computer technology to carefully target the cancer. Multiple radiation beams hit a tumor from several angles. A lower dose of radiation hits normal tissues, which results in less damage to healthy tissues.

Stereotactic Body Radiotherapy

Another form of radiation, *stereotactic body radiotherapy (SBRT),* is used for treating low-risk prostate cancer. High doses of radiation are delivered over a short period of time. The course of radiation can be given in one week, rather than up to forty-five treatments over seven to eight weeks with standard radiation. However,

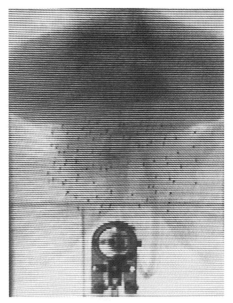

This X-ray was taken after brachytherapy, in which several dozen radioactive seeds were implanted in the prostate gland.

this radiation treatment is associated with more troublesome side effects, including inflammation of the urethra (tube that joins the bladder to the penis), incontinence, and blockage of the urinary tract.

Preparing for External Beam Radiation

Prior to starting treatments, you will have what is called a *simulation,* or planning session. At this time, a radiation oncologist outlines the radiation target—the area to which radiation beams will be aimed. A physicist develops a radiation treatment plan. The simulation process takes about twenty minutes.

You'll lie on a simulation couch—a narrow, rectangular table—and you will be injected with *iodine contrast material*. This material makes it possible for oncologists to view the prostate and internal tissues with a CT scan. The area to be treated will be drawn on your body with a marker, and you will receive tiny tattoos that mark the corners of the area to be treated.

Because it is important that you remain absolutely still during your treatments, an immobilization device will be used to hold your body in place. One of two types of devices may be used. One device is a bag containing a chemical that turns into Styrofoam and conforms to your shape. An alternative device is a bag filled with Styrofoam pellets that technicians use to form a body mold.

Undergoing External Beam Treatment

When it's time for your treatment, you'll be asked to empty your bladder. Then, you'll undress from the waist down, cover yourself with a gown or towel, and lie on a table. Radiation technicians will arrange your body to make sure the radiation is precisely focused.

You will not need any anesthesia. You will simply lie still while radiation beams are directed at your prostate and surrounding area. You will feel nothing on your skin during the treatment. You will hear a whirring noise, made by the linear accelerator, the machine most commonly used for external beam radiation; it moves around your body sending calculated doses of radiation to a tumor. The treatments last five minutes or less.

After External Beam Radiation

Because external beam radiation is not invasive, compared to brachytherapy, the recovery time is shorter than that for brachytherapy. As you enter the latter weeks of treatment, you might feel tired. Inflammation from radiation therapy releases chemicals into the bloodstream that can cause fatigue. It's also possible that some fatigue is associated with sleep deprivation that may result from the need to urinate frequently during the night; hormone-induced hot flashes may also cause sleep interruptions. These symptoms should subside shortly after treatment ends.

Combining Internal and External Radiation

Your doctor might recommend a combination of both internal and external radiation. External treatments can boost the radiation dosage delivered by brachytherapy—implanted seeds. Your doctor may recommend the combination treatment if there's a high risk of cancer outside the prostate but confined to the seminal vesicles and pelvic lymph nodes. Hormone therapy is often included in the combination treatment.

Are You a Candidate for Radiation Therapy?

Radiation treatment is best suited to men whose cancer is confined to the prostate. It can be a good alternative to surgery for older men or for those who may have other health considerations that prohibit them from having surgery.

External beam treatment is a better option than brachytherapy if you've had a *transurethral resection of the prostate (TURP)*. This procedure, for an enlarged prostate, "hollows out" the prostate, so there is usually not enough tissue to anchor the radioactive seeds. And because external beam therapy can be directed to the prostate, seminal vesicles, and pelvic lymph nodes, it can cover a larger area than seed implantation, which is usually restricted to the prostate itself.

A major consideration for undergoing external beam treatment is whether there is a treatment center near you, especially one that offers the three-dimensional conformal radiation or intensity-modulated radiation. If not, you may want to consider the time and expense involved in commuting to a regional center for two months. The typical radiation schedule is Monday through Friday for up to eight weeks. The daily treatment is part of what makes the treatment effective. You can't, for example, take a few weeks off in the middle of treatment.

Brachytherapy alone is usually recommended for those patients who are at low risk for recurrence. Patients with PSAs over 10, Gleason scores of 7 or above, and extensive cancers on both sides of the gland will usually be offered a combination of brachytherapy and external beam.

Radiation therapy is often not recommended for men who have large tumors or enlarged prostate glands. However, doctors may try to first shrink bulky prostate cancer tumors and the prostate itself with hormone therapy. Then, radiation treatments may be an option.

Side Effects of Radiation Therapy

Most men tolerate radiation therapy well. Lasting side effects are uncommon. The risk of death or life-threatening complications is very low with any form of radiation therapy. Still, it is important to be aware of potential side effects.

The conditions listed below may occur after brachytherapy or external beam radiation therapy. Whatever form of radiation you may have had, be sure to report all uncomfortable or alarming symptoms to your doctor, who may offer remedies.

Tenderness

Brachytherapy patients may be sore or have tenderness where brachytherapy needles were inserted. The soreness may also affect the testicles or penis; some men experience pain during ejaculation.

Skin Irritation

Skin in the treatment area may become red—like a sunburn. Or, the skin may become irritated, dry, and sensitive.

Incontinence

Severe incontinence occurs in fewer than 2 percent of men treated with radiation. Men who have undergone radiation treatment may have: urine leakage, frequent need to urinate, difficulty urinating, and stinging or burning during urination or bowel movements. You might see blood in your urine or semen. These problems will probably go away on their own within a few weeks after treatment, but be sure to mention them to your doctor.

If you should have a problem with urine retention, you'll feel bladder pressure but won't be able to urinate. Up to 15 percent of men require a Foley catheter during or after radiation. See chapter 7 for information on coping with incontinence.

Impotence

Radiation therapy affects a man's ability to get an erection. The risk of erectile dysfunction depends on several factors, including your age, overall health, having received hormonal therapy, and the type and dose of radiation given. Radiation may cause nerve damage in the pelvic area, restrict blood flow to the penis, or lower the level of testosterone. Also, the amount of semen ejaculated will decrease after radiation therapy.

Urethral Stricture

With radiation treatment, there is a slight risk of urethral stricture, a shrinking of the urethra caused by scar tissue. A physician can "stretch" the urethra back to size during an outpatient procedure.

Rectal Injury

Radiation treatment carries a risk of injury to the rectum. The first sign of such injury is often blood or mucus in the stool. Such an injury can be treated with laser surgery or with suppositories or enemas that contain cortisone.

You might also experience abdominal cramping and painful bowel movements.

Infection

Occasionally the prostate can become infected shortly after seed implantation; treatment typically calls for oral antibiotics.

Expelled Seeds

It is rare, but after brachytherapy, a radioactive seed may work its way out of the body during urination. This may happen if a seed has been dropped in the bladder; many doctors will check the bladder after seed implantation to make sure no seeds have been dropped. Your doctor will give you instructions on how to dispose of an expelled seed.

It is also possible that a seed could be passed during ejaculation. For this reason, it's recommended that you wear a condom during intercourse for several months after treatment.

Temporary Rise in PSA

More than a third of men treated with brachytherapy experience an increase in their PSA levels eight to ten months after radiation. This temporary PSA elevation is almost always due to prostate inflammation rather than recurrent prostate cancer.

Secondary Cancers

The risk is slight but it is possible to develop a secondary cancer in the area where radiation was delivered. The parts of the body mostly likely to be affected are the rectum and the bladder. If this were to occur, it could be years after the initial treatment. Talk to your physician about screening for such secondary cancers.

When to Seek Medical Attention

After radiation treatment, see your doctor or go to a hospital emergency room immediately if you have symptoms of inflammation or infection at an incision site—nausea, vomiting, fever of 100 degrees or higher, or chills.

After seed implantation, blood clots are less likely than after surgery, but there's a small chance of developing deep venous thrombosis (DVT)—blood clots that could travel from the legs to the lungs. Symptoms include pain or swelling in the legs, trouble breathing, or chest pain.

Also, see a doctor right away if you have blood or excessive mucus in your stool, if you experience severe pain, or if you are unable to urinate.

Follow-Up Care after Radiation

After radiation treatment for prostate cancer, follow-up care is important. You will see both your urologist and your radiation oncologist; they will want to manage any side effects you may be having. A follow-up care plan will include a digital rectal exam and PSA testing.

6 Chemotherapy

The role of chemotherapy in prostate cancer treatment is growing. Oncologists integrate chemotherapy into treatment plans for men with advanced or late-stage prostate cancer. Chemotherapy can slow the growth of cancer cells and control symptoms. It can extend life as well as improve quality of life.

How Chemotherapy Works

Chemotherapy agents are potent chemicals designed to kill cancer cells throughout the body. These agents work in various ways. Some prevent the growth of new blood vessels through which cancer can grow and spread. Others arrest cancer cells in different phases of their growth cycles. There are drugs that restore the normal cell "death process," which cancer cells resist. Still others attack cancer-cell genes to prevent cell growth and reproduction.

Historically, chemotherapy has had limited usefulness in treating prostate cancer. Because prostate cancer is slow growing, chemotherapy hasn't been practical for early-stage disease because it kills cells that are rapidly dividing. In addition, chemotherapy drugs travel through the body, destroying healthy and malignant cells alike and producing undesirable side effects.

Today, however, more-effective chemotherapeutic agents are available and doctors have more accurate ways to measure how well a chemotherapy agent is working.

At the same time, there are better medications to treat side effects.

When Is Chemotherapy Recommended?

Chemotherapy is a treatment option for a diagnosis of metastatic castration-resistant prostate cancer, the most challenging form of advanced prostate cancer. Doctors typically use chemotherapy only when a man is having significant symptoms, such as bone pain and urinary problems.

Chemotherapy Drugs for Advanced Prostate Cancer

When chemotherapy is called for, oncologists prescribe from a class of drugs called *taxoids*. These drugs prevent cancer-cell division by interfering with the internal structures of cells, causing them to die. If one drug is not effective, an oncologist may choose another drug.

Preparing for Chemotherapy

Before chemotherapy, patients sometimes have blood tests, X-rays and other imaging studies (scans), and biopsies. These tests help doctors locate metastases and determine whether the patient is a good candidate for chemotherapy. Patients in satisfactory health when chemotherapy begins are less likely than others to experience troublesome side effects.

Necessary dental work should be completed at least two weeks before treatments start. Having dental work during the course of chemotherapy is risky because chemotherapy patients are vulnerable to infection and mouth sores. (Chemotherapy kills healthy fast-growing cells such as those in the lining of the mouth.)

Days or weeks before surgery, doctors may start patients on antinausea drugs and advise them to stay well hydrated by drinking water and to avoid spicy and fatty foods. Note that you will likely be advised to not eat or drink fluids for at least two hours before a chemotherapy treatment.

Receiving Chemotherapy

Chemotherapy is given intravenously (IV) in cycles, meaning a treatment is given and then it is followed by a recovery period. Then, the next treatment is given and is followed by a recovery period. Treatments are given in cycles because chemotherapy kills cancer cells that are rapidly dividing but doesn't affect those cells that are at rest. Repeated cycles improve the odds of finding and destroying cancer cells when they are in the reproduction phase. Time off between treatments also allows normal tissues to recover. Chemotherapy may be administered once a week, but once every three weeks is usual. For advanced prostate cancer, chemotherapy may continue as long as it is working and side effects are well tolerated.

Chemotherapy by injection or IV drip *(infusion)* typically takes place in a clinic or hospital. Each treatment may take a few minutes to several hours, depending on the drug, the dose, and the delivery method. Doctors admit some chemotherapy patients to the hospital for overnight observation after the first treatment.

Slow-growing prostate cancer cells require longer exposure to cancer-fighting chemicals than do fast-growing cells. Frequent low doses tend to be more comfortable for patients, and may be more effective than fewer, larger doses.

Some chemotherapy drugs are given in pill form and can be taken at home.

What Is a PICC Line?

One way of giving chemotherapy at frequent low doses is through a *peripherally inserted central catheter (PICC) line.* Similar to an IV, a PICC line is a long, thin, flexible plastic tube through which medication is delivered and blood samples can be drawn. The PICC remains in

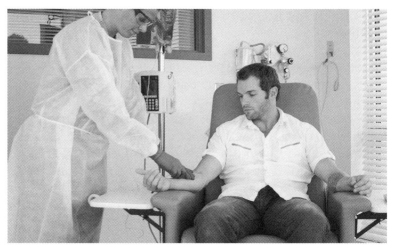

Chemotherapy is given in cycles, usually three weeks apart. This approach gives healthy cells that are affected by the treatment time to recover.

place throughout the course of treatment so there's no need for a needle stick at every treatment. PICC also greatly reduces the risk of tissue damage that may occur when chemotherapy drugs leak into nearby tissues during a needle infusion. If such injury does occur, a doctor can prescribe a cream to rub onto the injured area.

The PICC is inserted with a simple surgical procedure. After applying a local anesthetic, a doctor or specially trained nurse inserts the PICC line, usually in the upper arm. The tube is carefully threaded through the body into a large vein next to the heart where blood flow quickly distributes medication throughout the body. Patients need to be careful that the insertion site remains covered, clean, and dry.

Discontinuing Chemotherapy

In some cases, an oncologist may recommend discontinuing chemotherapy or they may want to switch to a different drug. In making this choice, oncologists generally consider three factors:

- *Is the patient handling the chemotherapy well?* Doctors monitor a patient's side effects and overall condition, determining whether the patient remains well enough to tolerate and benefit from the drugs.
- *Is the chemotherapy working?* The doctor performs tests for evidence that the drug is working.
- *Are there serious adverse side effects after chemotherapy?* If the medication seems to cause severe side effects, such as liver toxicity or a dramatic drop in white blood cells, a patient and their oncologist may decide to discontinue chemotherapy, at least temporarily. At this point, the optimal choice may be pain medication to keep the patient comfortable.

In some cases, oncologists have the option of switching to a different chemotherapy agent, especially if a drug is causing serious side effects or if an agent doesn't appear to be working well.

Side Effects of Chemotherapy

Chemotherapy affects cells throughout the entire body, including healthy tissues, and this produces side effects. The drugs target primarily rapidly dividing cells, such as those in bone marrow, hair follicles, and the reproductive and digestive systems; this is why individuals on chemotherapy will have side effects such as hair loss and nausea. Side effects differ with different drugs. When anticipating side effects, remember:

- Not everyone experiences every side effect. The dose, frequency, and duration of chemotherapy makes a difference in side effects.
- Side effects usually resolve when the body has a chance to recover after chemotherapy.

- There are a number of chemotherapy drugs to choose from, so if one is particularly troublesome, another may be better tolerated.

Side effects can be alleviated with prescription drugs, over-the-counter products, lifestyle adjustments, and other strategies. It's important to mention side effects to your medical oncologist as soon as they occur so they can be quickly treated. The following side effects are possible.

Fatigue

One of the most common side effects of chemotherapy is fatigue, often brought on by a low red blood cell count, called *anemia.* Red blood cells deliver oxygen throughout the body. Inadequate oxygen supplies in tissues and organs cause fatigue. Severe anemia during chemotherapy can be treated with a blood transfusion or a medication that stimulates production of red blood cells. Here are a few tips for coping with fatigue:

- Limit activities; do only those things that are most important.
- Take several short naps or breaks during the day.
- Try taking short walks or exercising lightly.
- Maintain good nutrition; try to eat a well-balanced diet.

For some patients, fatigue occurs soon after treatment. Others feel fatigued during the entire course of therapy or beyond, even after chemotherapy has ended. It can take weeks for your energy to return to normal. For active patients, fatigue can be a source of frustration, even depression. Look for ways to remain positive and remember that the fatigue is temporary.

Stomach Irritation

Chemotherapy can cause a variety of side effects throughout the digestive tract. Common side effects include nausea, vomiting, constipation, diarrhea, and loss of appetite.

Irritation of the stomach and intestinal lining can cause diarrhea and abdominal cramping lasting several hours to several days. With severe diarrhea there is a risk of dehydration and loss of nutrients. If you have severe dehydration, you may be hospitalized for intravenous fluid replacement.

Here are suggestions for avoiding intestinal problems:

- If recommended by your doctor, drink at least six to eight glasses of water daily.
- Avoid high-fiber, greasy, rich, and spicy foods; any food high in sugar; caffeinated drinks; and alcohol.
- Eat small amounts of solid food frequently throughout the day.
- Eat and drink slowly; chew foods well.
- Suck on ice cubes, mints, or ginger candies (unless prevented by mouth sores).

Check with your doctor before using over-the-counter products such as Imodium-AD for diarrhea or milk of magnesia for constipation. There are prescription drugs available for these conditions.

Diarrhea, vomiting, and inability to eat can be dangerous, causing you to become malnourished or dehydrated. Report these conditions to your doctor. Don't assume they're just part of the treatment process.

Mouth Sores

Mouth and throat sores can be aggravated both by a low white-blood-cell count and by chemotherapy's effects on your digestive system. Mouth sores are less common with chemotherapy for prostate cancer than for other cancers, but they can arise with any chemotherapy.

Mouth sores emerge as painful lesions or ulcers on the lips, in the mouth, on the gums, or inside the throat.

Mouth sores may be very uncomfortable and may make eating and drinking difficult. The sores can also become infected.

If you develop mouth sores, ask your doctor about medication to treat them. Here are other ways to deal with mouth sores:

- Brush and floss your teeth often, using a soft-bristle brush to avoid irritating gums.
- Avoid mouthwashes that contain alcohol. Some doctors recommend rinsing your mouth with a mild saltwater solution (but other doctors claim that salt can worsen mouth sores, so ask your doctor).
- Stay hydrated by drinking plenty of water.
- Suck on ice chips; they may be soothing.
- Eat soft foods, such as baby food, cooled oatmeal, mashed vegetables, yogurt, ice cream, milk shakes, and smoothies. Avoid hard, crunchy foods and those with high acid content (tomatoes, citrus fruits) or high in salt or spices, and caffeine.
- Don't smoke or chew tobacco.

Nerve Pain

Chemotherapy may cause nerve pain, called *neuropathy*. Symptoms may include weakness, numbness, tingling sensation, or pain. Neuropathy commonly occurs in the hands and feet, but it may also occur in the mouth, throat, or chest. An individual may also feel abnormal tongue sensations, a choking sensation, or pressure on the chest.

The severity of nerve pain depends on how much of a chemotherapy agent you received and the length of time it was given. Report any pain or tingling to your oncologist right away so that he or she can adjust or suspend treatment.

Neuropathy may be either acute or chronic. Acute neuropathy goes away within days after a chemotherapy treatment, while chronic neuropathy can persist for weeks to months. Symptoms may be constant, or they may come and go. The chronic form of neuropathy can become irreversible if chemotherapy treatment continues. An oncologist may reduce the chemotherapy dose or stop the treatment altogether.

Folic acid, one of the B vitamins, has been shown in numerous studies to be effective against chemotherapy-induced neuropathy. Medications are also available to alleviate neuropathy pain.

Infections

Chemotherapy can damage the bone marrow, where blood cells originate. Up to 70 percent of circulating white blood cells, called *neutrophils,* destroy bacteria in the blood. A neutrophil deficiency, called *neutropenia,* compromises the immune system. Because the immune system wards off disease, a weakened immune system makes one prone to infections and pneumonia.

Be alert for signs of infection—fever over 100 degrees, shaking, chills, or sweats; coughing up dark or bloody sputum; pain or burning with urination; and pain or redness around incisions or cuts. To reduce your risk of infection, take these precautions:

- Wash your hands often during the day, especially after using the bathroom.
- Avoid anyone who has a cold, flu, measles, or chicken pox.
- Stay away from children who have recently received vaccinations.
- Clean cuts and scrapes right away.
- Wear gloves when gardening or cleaning up after pets or children.

- Use a soft toothbrush that won't hurt your gums.
- Clean yourself thoroughly after each bowel movement; if the area around your anus becomes irritated or if you have hemorrhoids, notify your doctor.

If you have symptoms of infection, seek medical attention immediately. Infections can be effectively treated with antibiotics.

Impaired Blood Clotting

Chemotherapy can cause a condition called *thrombo-cytopenia,* caused by a low blood platelet count. Platelets are blood cells that help with clotting. Mild thrombocytopenia may produce no symptoms. A severe deficiency of platelets may show up in a purplish rash on the hands and feet or may cause easy bruising; these symptoms would indicate bleeding under the skin. Spontaneous nosebleeds may occur. In serious cases, internal bleeding may occur.

Because there are no specific medications for impaired blood clotting, an oncologist will usually delay or suspend chemotherapy when a patient's blood platelet count is low. This break in treatment gives the platelet count time to rise on its own. If the platelet count drops dangerously, however, a blood platelet transfusion may be needed to avoid bleeding complications.

Throughout your treatment, your doctor will monitor your blood counts. After the course of chemotherapy has ended, you may receive treatment for low blood platelets.

Hair and Nail Changes

Some chemotherapy patients never have problems with their hair or nails. However, most experience at least some changes. Because hair and fingernails are made up of rapidly reproducing cells, they are affected by chemotherapy which kills fast-growing cells. Although hair loss can occur anywhere on the body, it is mainly confined to the head. Your fingernails may become brittle and develop ridges in them. Little can be done to prevent chemotherapy-induced hair loss. There are no drugs, food supplements, or products that can prevent it. Still, here are tips for coping with hair loss.

- Use mild shampoos.
- Use a soft hairbrush.
- Use low heat on your hair dryer.
- Don't dye your hair.
- Protect your scalp from the sun with a hat or sunscreen.

After chemotherapy is completed, these scalp cells usually recover and hair will regrow, and nails will go back to normal.

Skin Changes

During chemotherapy, your skin may be itchy and dry. You might develop a rash, sores, or even blisters. Be sure to let your doctor know if these conditions are severe because skin abnormalities can signal an allergic reaction to chemotherapy drugs. To prevent infection, immediately call your doctor's attention to any open sores on your skin.

Take warm but not hot showers and baths. Baking soda in your bathwater can soothe itching. Ask your doctor about taking vitamin E or zinc supplements. Your doctor might also recommend skin products containing aloe vera. Use mild skin cleansers, shampoos, and laundry products (such as Dreft and Ivory Snow) that are gentle enough for sensitive skin. Drink plenty of fluids to hydrate your skin, and avoid extremes of heat or cold.

You'll probably be susceptible to sunburn so be sure to wear sunscreen, at least 15 SPF, any time you go outdoors.

Nervous System Changes

Some chemotherapy drugs can damage the nervous system and may have an effect on brain functions. Tell your doctor immediately about symptoms such as headache, confusion, depression, fever, numbness or tingling in the extremities, dry mouth, vision problems, and ringing in the ears. Prescription medication may prevent many of these problems. For example, antidepressants may help with depression.

Another possible impairment, "brain fog," refers to feeling confused or having problems concentrating. This symptom is usually mild, but may linger from months to years. The severity of it depends on how much chemotherapy was given and the length of time it was given. If you find yourself having memory and thinking impairments, here are steps you can take:

- Keep a notepad handy to jot down reminders to yourself.
- Keep a calendar nearby for scheduling appointments and events.
- Get plenty of rest.
- Ask for support from family members and friends.

Some patients report that exercise, music therapy, art, or reading helps them deal with memory and thinking impairments.

Kidney and Liver Damage

A few chemotherapy drugs may cause liver or kidney damage, which can sometimes be prevented with prescription drugs. Regular blood tests monitor kidney and liver function. If damage is suspected, a different chemotherapy drug may be used.

Directed Immunotherapy

A newer type of treatment, *directed immunotherapy,* is used to treat *metastatic castration-resistant prostate cancer.* This cancer occurs when malignant cells continue growing despite previous surgery, radiation, or drug therapy to suppress male hormones.

Immunotherapy is not actually a form of chemotherapy, but, like chemotherapy, it circulates through the entire body. The drug is designed to jump-start your own immune system so it can better fight cancer. If you are to receive such a drug, it will be tailored specifically for you. First, your own immune cells are extracted from your blood. Then, in a lab, the cells are stimulated to fight cancer cells. The drug, containing these immune cells, is then given back to you through an intravenous infusion. You will likely receive three treatments that are each two weeks apart.

Side effects are typically limited to the first few days after treatment. These side effects may include feeling as if you have a flu, with fever, chills, nausea, and muscle aches.

Follow-Up Care after Chemotherapy

After you complete your chemotherapy, you will see your urologist and medical oncologist for follow-up examinations. You'll have blood tests, X-rays, and scans. Your oncologist will also monitor any side effects that may linger.

The frequency of such visits are determined by the nature of your treatment and your overall health.

7 Life after Prostate Cancer

If you're in the process of undergoing cancer treatment or if you're recovering from treatment, you may not be feeling like yourself. Along with your loved ones, you have been through a cancer diagnosis and this can take an emotional toll.

In addition to healing physically, be sure to take care of your emotional needs as well. You may be feeling lonely or depressed, or both. Remember, avenues of help are available, whether it be physical, emotional, or spiritual.

Coping Emotionally

Many men with prostate cancer find it difficult to ask for support. But, think of all the emotional support you've offered others throughout your life. Now, it's time for you to receive support. There are a number of things you can do to help you cope emotionally during or after cancer treatment. And remember, part of being independent is knowing when to ask for help.

Support Groups

Some of the most powerful support available comes from support groups made up of men who are prostate cancer survivors. These men gather in community centers and hospital meeting rooms, or in online discussion groups. They share their stories, draw strength from each other, and learn about advances in prostate cancer treatment. They know what you've been through. In addition to emotional support, they can recommend physicians, therapists, books, and other resources.

There's at least one more good reason to get involved with a support group. Studies have consistently shown that cancer patients in strong support groups live longer. "Strong" is a key word here. Find a support group that is upbeat and encouraging. If you visit a group several times and don't feel emotionally nourished, that particular group may not be right for you. Every group has its own "personality." Seek one that is a good fit for you.

How do you find a support group? First, ask a member of your medical team. Also, see the Resources section in the back of this book.

Spiritual Resources

Some men gain a sense of well-being in prayer or fellowship groups, meditation, or yoga classes. Through the ages, people have relied on prayer, pastoral counseling, and close-knit religious communities to help them through illness and other difficulties. Many members of the clergy in nearly every denomination have received training in pastoral counseling.

Help for Depression

It's not uncommon for men to become depressed when they are diagnosed with prostate cancer. Depression can often occur after treatment. Men often feel encouraged by medical staff during visits to the clinic for treatments; however, after treatments end, it's common to experience a "letdown," when you're no longer seeing medical staff regularly. Don't delay getting help for depression or anxiety. Talk to your doctor. With medication, counseling, or a combination of the two, you can find the tools that are important right now for taking care of yourself. A positive outlook is your best friend.

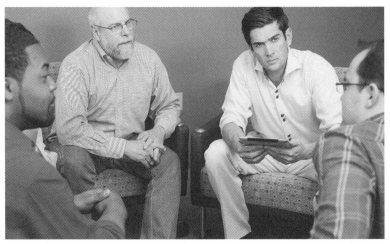

Prostate cancer support groups can offer powerful emotional support during and after treatment.

Talk to Your Partner

If you have a partner, hopefully you have their emotional support and can share your fears as well as your joys. Or, perhaps you have a close friend or relative you can count on to be there for you. Maybe you're a person who has held things in all your life. Perhaps you've thought that being "strong" meant dealing with your problems on your own. It's time to let down your defenses and seek support.

Realize that your prostate cancer affects your loved ones almost as much as it affects you, even if none of you talk about it. Often, communicating openly with trusted friends and loved ones can help each of you to emerge stronger than you were before. This is an opportunity for your relationships to grow.

Your Children, Family Members, Friends, and Coworkers

What should you tell the kids? Many counselors recommend a balance between honesty and reassurance, depending on your children's ages. Grown children are likely to feel hurt if they're deprived of a chance to help and support their dad, and even very young children can sense something upsetting is going on, and they may become anxious. They, too, will need assurance.

What you say to other people depends on your relationship with them and their need to know. Don't worry that you're burdening people when you tell them about your illness. Most people are eager to help when they can, even if it's just by listening.

When people ask how they can help, tell them. Do you need transportation to the doctor's office or the hospital? Do you just want someone to talk to? Let them know. If they genuinely care about you, you'll be doing them a favor by letting them contribute to your well-being.

Your Doctor Can Help

Your doctor and his or her staff can give you information, referrals, and encouragement. Be assured that your physicians have treated hundreds of other prostate cancer patients. Perhaps you can alleviate anxiety by asking questions. These doctors understand the fears and concerns that men have. They are used to questions such as "What kind of undergarment is best for leakage?" and "What can I do for impotence?" By being completely honest with your doctor, you may learn about a drug or procedure that could improve the quality of your life.

Coping with Incontinence

Some degree of incontinence is likely after radical prostatectomy or radiation therapy. It's almost always temporary, though in some cases it can be a problem lasting years. In fact, after radiation therapy, incontinence may get worse over time because radiation-damaged cells can't repair themselves as other cells do.

Bladder control depends on the *urinary sphincter* muscles around the urethra. Prostate surgery or radiation can damage or weaken these muscles so that they no longer keep urine from leaking out of the bladder. As mentioned earlier, this type of incontinence is called *stress incontinence;* it is the leaking of urine when you cough, sneeze, laugh, or get out of a chair.

Less common is *urge incontinence*—you have the urge to urinate, but feel as if you can't get to the bathroom in time. *Overflow incontinence* occurs when normal urine flow is blocked and the bladder is always full. There are several treatments for incontinence that could be a fit for you.

Monitor Fluid Intake

After your initial treatment, don't drink more than two quarts of water a day, and limit caffeine and alcohol to avoid undue stress on the new connection between your bladder and your urethra. Ask your doctor when this connection is likely to be fully healed. Discuss water intake with your doctor because you also want to avoid becoming dehydrated.

Medications for Incontinence

Drugs are usually the first line of defense in treating incontinence. Depending on the type of incontinence you have, your doctor might prescribe simple decongestants or antidepressants; these drugs help tighten urethra muscles. Other types of drugs are also available to treat incontinence.

Exercises for Incontinence

One of the best ways to overcome or diminish the incontinence problem is with *Kegel exercises,* also called *pelvic floor exercises.* These exercises are so simple you can do them almost anywhere. Simply tighten your pelvic muscles, keep them tight for about ten seconds, and then release.

You use your pelvic muscles many times a day. They're the muscles you tighten to keep from urinating before you can get to the bathroom. To practice, try stopping the urine stream after you've begun urinating. Some doctors tell patients to practice tightening and releasing their muscles over a five-minute period, two to three times each day. You can start these exercises before prostate cancer treatment. After you've completed treatment, continue this regimen until you're no longer troubled with incontinence.

Your doctor may refer you to physical therapy for help rehabilitating your pelvic muscles. You might think Kegel exercises would not be difficult to master, but it's surprisingly easy to do them wrong. It's important to tighten only the pelvic muscles, not the buttocks or the abdominal or thigh muscles.

Male Sling

For this procedure, a strip of abdominal or synthetic tissue is surgically placed in the pelvis to compress the urethra and stop leakage. The procedure can usually be done on an outpatient basis in less than half an hour. It requires only a two-inch incision between the scrotum and the rectum. Studies have shown improvement in 80 percent of the men treated.

Condom Catheter

A *condom catheter* is a device that drains leaked urine from the penis. The condom, usually latex, is attached to the penis with adhesive. A plastic tube connects the condom catheter to a bag taped to the leg. The urine stays in the attached bag until it is emptied.

If you are allergic to latex, the condom catheter probably isn't for you. Many doctors recommend against the device for other reasons as well. You may be tempted to rely on the condom catheter rather than work to regain urinary control. Also, this device may contribute to urinary tract infections and other problems. If you do use the condom catheter, do so for only brief travels outside your home; the bag must be emptied every thirty minutes.

Penile Clamp

An external *penile clamp* (called a *Cunningham clamp*) can be effective in controlling incontinence. The device, which has a soft foam inside, is placed half way down the penis shaft; when in place and closed, it compresses the urethra so that urine cannot escape. When used as prescribed, the clamp is safe and convenient. This inexpensive device is available from your urologist.

Artificial Urinary Sphincter

If you have lingering incontinence, your physician may suggest an *artificial urinary sphincter;* this device has three parts: a silicon rubber cuff that fits around the urethra, a balloon that is placed in your lower abdomen, and an inflatable pump in the scrotum. Having the device inserted involves a surgical procedure, which is done on an outpatient basis or with an overnight hospital stay.

When the cuff contains fluid, it compresses the urethra so that urine can't escape. When you want to urinate, you squeeze the pump a few times. Activating the pump causes the fluid to flow from the cuff to the balloon. After you urinate, the fluid will flow back into the cuff. When you squeeze the pump, it causes urine to flow from the cuff into the balloon. By emptying the cuff, the urethra opens and you can urinate. Then, the cuff re-inflates.

The procedure is successful up to 90 percent of the time and carries minimal risk. As with any minor surgery, there's a slight chance of bleeding or infection. Rare complications can include urinary retention and malfunction or breakage of the device.

Collagen Injections

Collagen is a natural protein that's commonly used in cosmetic procedures to plump up facial skin and diminish fine lines and wrinkles. The same principle applies in this simple outpatient procedure. When collagen is injected into the tissues around the bladder neck, they swell to prevent urine leakage out of the bladder. Only men with mild incontinence benefit from collagen injections, which have to be repeated—two or three times initially and again if the leakage comes back. The procedure can remain effective from months to several years.

Your doctor will do a skin test to make sure you're not allergic to the collagen, which is derived from cattle. This is a very important precaution, as an allergic reaction could be life threatening. If you've had a radical prostatectomy followed by radiation therapy, collagen injections will not work for you; the injections can't "bulk up" the radiation-treated bladder neck.

Incontinence Undergarments

In every drugstore, you'll find shelves with a variety of disposable pads and underpants for adults with incontinence. Some are made specifically for men. They're very useful, even necessary, immediately after a radical prostatectomy. Ask your doctor to recommend a product. Change your pad or undergarment often to avoid odor and chafing.

Coping with Impotence

Every medical treatment for prostate cancer carries a risk of temporary or permanent impotence. It's impossible to know before treatment which men will become impotent and for how long. Even among men in their forties who have the nerve-sparing radical prostatectomy, 10 percent are impotent afterward.

Normally, when you start to get an erection, blood flows into the chambers in the penis. It is the blood in these chambers that keeps the penis erect. While you're aroused, the blood vessels are sealed off and the blood can't flow back out. This natural process may not work well, or at all, after prostate cancer treatment.

During prostate surgery or radiation, blood vessels and nerve pathways to the penis may be damaged, causing impotence. Hormone therapy causes impotence in an entirely different way, by eliminating production of testosterone, the hormone that governs male sexuality. During hormone therapy for prostate cancer, men not only become impotent, they lose interest in sex. Potency may return when treatment stops.

Impotence in Men

With or without prostate cancer, 25 percent of men will experience some level of impotence by age sixty-five. Impotence can be a result from diabetes, hypertension, and other disorders, or from medications, alcohol, smoking, and psychological conditions.

Keep in mind that the word "impotence" refers only to the inability to have an erection. Other facets of sexual activity— desire, ejaculation, and orgasm—are separate matters. Even with impotence, you can usually still enjoy sexual activity and experience orgasms.

Talk to Your Partner

You may find it most helpful to communicate openly with your partner. Talk about your feelings associated with impotence. You may feel sad, discouraged, or even embarrassed. You're not alone. Many men go through these feelings. Honest communication will help you emotionally. And, you can experiment with techniques you both find enjoyable, whether or not they produce an erection.

Drugs for Impotence

Your doctor might prescribe oral medications such as Viagra, Levitra, or Cialis for erectile dysfunction. These drugs work by blocking an enzyme found in penile tissues. When the enzyme is blocked, the smooth muscles of the penis can relax to allow blood to flow in.

Most men tolerate these drugs well, but there are some men who should never take them. If you have coronary

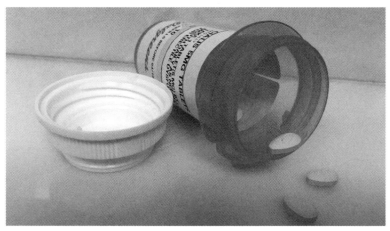

Drugs such as Viagra, Cialis, and Levitra increase blood flow to the penis, creating an erection. However, the drugs do not simulate arousal.

artery disease, get clearance from your cardiologist before using one of these drugs. If you're taking medicine containing nitrates (such as nitroglycerine or isosorbides), drugs for erectile dysfunction are not recommended. The combination of drugs may cause a dangerous drop in blood pressure.

It is uncommon for these drugs to cause side effects; however, they may cause headache, indigestion, runny nose, diarrhea, dizziness, and vision disturbances such as temporarily seeing a blue haze. Another possible side effect is flushing—a reddening of the skin with a sensation of being hot.

Note that these drugs to help men achieve erections are not aphrodisiacs. They won't help you become aroused, but will help you achieve an erection.

Injections for Impotence

If you have taken erectile dysfunction drugs for two to four months after surgery, but are still unable to achieve an erection, your doctor may recommend *penile injection therapy*. These injections use a very fine needle. You can give them yourself, and they are painless and effective.

Penile Pump

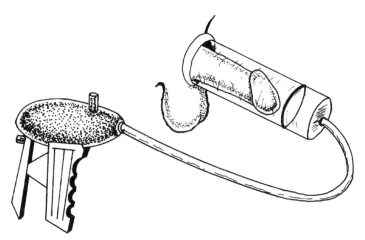

A penile pump is used externally to make blood flow into the shaft and tip of the penis, causing an erection.

The injections contain a drug called a *vasodilator;* it widens blood vessels in the penis shaft. As the blood vessels open, the smooth muscles relax in the penis. Then, within ten to twenty minutes, both chambers of the penis fill with blood, giving you an erection that lasts for thirty minutes to two hours.

It's important that you take the lowest effective dose possible. If the dose is too high, you could have a prolonged erection that could actually become dangerous—the trapped blood loses oxygen and can cause tissue damage in the penis.

Side effects can include small blood clots, burning sensation after the injection, damage to the urethra, and a fibrous tissue buildup in the penis. Infection should not be a problem if you keep the injection site clean.

You may have heard about men who use testosterone injections to restore sexual function, but be assured that no doctor will prescribe testosterone for you if you are at risk for prostate cancer or are being treated for it. As

Penile Implant

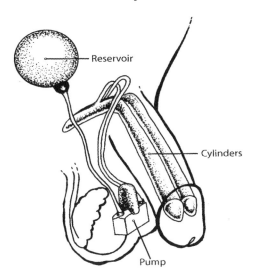

Reservoir

Cylinders

Pump

Penile implants are a consideration if other measures fail to produce erections. Long-term data shows penile implants to be highly effective and reliable.

explained earlier, testosterone can stimulate the growth of prostate cancer.

Vacuum Erection Devices

A *vacuum erection device* is an airtight tube that you place over your lubricated penis. Pumping the device creates a vacuum that draws blood into your penis. The pump has a rubber ring that slides off the pump and onto the base of the penis; this keeps the blood from flowing back out. These rings come in different sizes. If you have the correct size ring, it won't be uncomfortable.

Vacuum erection devices are safe and effective. You can use them as often as you like, but you must remove the ring after thirty minutes to restore normal blood flow.

Penile Implants

A *penile implant* is a consideration if other measures fail to produce erections. An implant, which is inflatable, is surgically inserted, typically through a small incision in the scrotum. The device has two cylinders that are placed in the penis shaft and a fluid reservoir that is placed in the lower abdomen; a small pump is placed in the scrotum.

To achieve an erection, a man squeezes the pump by hand, the fluid in the reservoir is released into the two cylinders, and the penis becomes erect. After sexual activity, a man presses the pump; this allows the fluid to backfill into the reservoir, and the two cylinders deflate.

The procedure to insert an implant can be performed on an outpatient basis or with an overnight stay in the hospital. There are slight risks of infection, scarring, or damage to the two natural chambers that run the length of the penis. Research shows that 91 percent of men are satisfied with their implants.

If Cancer Recurs

Anyone who has had cancer knows what it's like to worry about a recurrence. For a while at least, every symptom can set alarm bells ringing. You don't want to live in a state of heightened anxiety, but you're wise to check with your doctor when your body sends you signals you don't understand.

By testing your blood regularly, your doctor will be alert to any PSA increase. If your PSA continues to rise, it *may* indicate that cancer has returned. If cancer does recur, there are treatment options.

Salvage Therapy

If you should have a recurrence of cancer, your urologist may recommend what's called *salvage therapy*. Salvage treatments may be given in the hope that a cure is still possible, especially if the recurrence is confined to the prostate area. Otherwise, salvage treatments can prolong life by controlling the cancer.

Only certain salvage therapies can be tried when other treatments have failed. For example, it's unlikely that your physician would recommend surgery to remove the prostate gland after radiation treatments failed. Prostate removal at this point would probably not remove all the cancer, and is associated with severe side effects and complications.

The most commonly used salvage treatment is radiation, especially for men with a recurrence of cancer in the bed of the prostate gland after surgical removal. External radiation may also be used for recurrence after brachytherapy, although it carries an increased risk of irritation or damage to both the urethra and the rectum.

Radioactive seed implantation is seldom used as salvage therapy. It is effective only if cancer is confined to the prostate gland. Otherwise, there is often no good way to anchor the seeds.

If your primary treatment was internal or external radiation, your doctor may want to start hormone therapy. Hormone treatments probably won't eliminate cancer altogether, but the treatment can prolong your life and improve your quality of life for many years. Another form of salvage treatment includes cryoablation, in which tissues are frozen.

It is not unheard of for a man to undergo salvage surgery to remove the prostate gland, but the operation can be risky. The odds are increased for severe incontinence and impotence. There is also risk of injury to the rectal wall, and a man might require a permanent colostomy. A colostomy involves a surgical procedure in which the large intestine is routed to an external bag, where fecal waste collects.

Palliative Care

If cancer cannot be stopped from spreading, an oncologist may suggest palliative care. The purpose of this treatment is to keep patients as comfortable as possible. One such treatment, spot radiation, is localized external beam radiation therapy used to treat pain or to shrink tumors. Spot radiation can also prevent a tumor from causing pressure on the spinal cord. Such pressure is a serious condition that, if untreated, can lead to paralysis.

Injections of radioactive materials also target cancer in the bones and provide relief for up to six months. These injections can create a drop in blood production in the bone marrow; this may require blood transfusions.

Other treatments may include over-the-counter painkillers as well as prescription painkillers. In cases of severe back pain, your physician may recommend surgery to alleviate pressure caused by a pinched nerve in the spine.

In Closing

Whether you've just been diagnosed with prostate cancer or you've begun treatment, I hope you find this book helpful. By being knowledgeable about prostate cancer and its treatment, you can make more-informed decisions.

Life expectancy for men with prostate cancer continues to rise, in large part because of early detection. When I first began practice as a urologist in 1984, we found prostate cancer that had spread in 40 percent of men when they were diagnosed. Now, men with metastatic disease make up less than 5 percent of new cases. Not only has early detection increased, but we've made improvements to all approaches to prostate cancer treatment—surgery, radiation, hormonal therapy, and chemotherapy.

After you complete treatment, your doctors will monitor you closely at first. If you are doing well after completing treatment, you will require less frequent follow-up.

A cancer diagnosis carries with it a significant emotional impact. I hope you will seek the emotional support you need—it will help you heal. Wherever you are in your journey through prostate cancer, I wish you the very best.

Appendix

Simplified Summary of TNM Staging System for Prostate Cancer

The staging system below is used by physicians to describe how far a cancer has spread. The most commonly used staging system is the American Joint Committee on Cancer's "TNM System." The system will appear complex to many readers. Ask your urologist to explain how your cancer is being staged with this system.

T = Tumor **N** = Nodes **M** = Metastases

Stage T1

Tumor is microscopic and confined to prostate but is undetectable by a digital rectal exam (DRE) or by ultrasound. Usually discovered by PSA tests or biopsies.

Stage T2

Tumor is confined to prostate and can be detected by DRE or ultrasound.

Stage T3 or T4

In stage T3, the cancer has spread to tissue adjacent to the prostate or to the seminal vesicles. Stage T4 tumors have spread to organs near the prostate, such as the bladder.

Stage N+ or M+

Cancer has spread to pelvic lymph nodes (N+) or to lymph nodes, organs, or bones distant from the prostate (M+).

Expanded Summary of Staging Systems	Whitmore-Jewett System	TNM System
In the earliest stage, prostate cancer can't be felt during a DRE. It is said to be found "incidentally" during BPH surgery. Biopsied tissue at this stage is less than 5 percent cancerous. Because it is confined to the prostate, small, and low-grade, some doctors recommend "watchful waiting" rather than curative treatment.	A1	T1a
The cancer is not *palpable* (it can't be felt during a DRE) and is found incidentally, during BPH surgery. More than 5 percent of the biopsied tissue is cancerous.	A2	T1b
The cancer is not palpable, but the PSA is elevated and cancer may be found in samples from a needle biopsy.	A3	T1c
Cancer is felt during DRE but is a small nodule confined to less than half of one side of the prostate.	B1N	T2a
Cancer is palpable during DRE and is found in more than half of one side.	B2	T2c
Cancer occupies one side and is growing outside the capsule.	C1	T3a
Cancer is in both sides and is growing outside the prostate.	C1	T3c
Cancer has spread to the seminal vesicles.	C2	T3c
Cancer has spread to the bladder neck, rectum, or external sphincter, or all three.	C2	T4a
Cancer has spread to other areas in the pelvis.	C2	T4b
There is no cancer found in the lymph nodes.	—	N0
2 cm or a smaller amount of cancer has spread to lymph nodes.	D1	N1 (N+)
2 to 5 cm of cancer has spread to lymph nodes.	D1	N2 (N+)
5 cm or a greater amount of cancer has spread to lymph nodes.	D1	N3 (N+)

Expanded Summary of Staging Systems	Whitmore-Jewett System	TNM System
Cancer has not spread beyond pelvic tissues and lymph nodes.	—	M0
Cancer has metastasized beyond the pelvis to bones and perhaps other areas.	D2	M1 (M+)

Resources

American Brachytherapy Society (ABS)
11130 Sunrise Valley Drive, Suite 350
Reston, VA 20191
Phone: (703) 234-4078
www.americanbrachytherapy.org

American Cancer Society
15999 Clifton Road NE
Atlanta, GA 30329-4251
Phone: (800) 227-2345
www.cancer.org

American Urological Association
1000 Corporate Boulevard
Linthicum, MD 21090
Phone: (800) 828-7866
www.urologyhealth.org

Cancer Care, Inc.
275 Seventh Avenue
New York, NY 10001
Phone: (800) 813-HOPE
www.cancercare.org

National Cancer Institute
NCI Office of Communications and Education
Public Inquiries Office
9609 Medicate Center Drive
Bethesda, MD 20892
Phone: (800) 422-6237)
www.nci.nih.gov

National Coalition for Cancer Survivorship
8455 Colesvile Road, Suite 930
Silver Spring, MD 20910
Phone: (888) 650-9127
www.canceradvocacy.org

National Comprehensive Cancer Network
275 Commerce Drive, Suite 300
Fort Washington, PA 19034
Phone: (215) 690-0300
ww.nccn.com

The New Prostate Cancer InfoLink
P.O. Box 66355
Virginia Beach, VA 23466,
http://prostatecancerinfolink.net

Patient Advocates for Advance Cancer Treatments (PAACT)
P.O. Box 45
Sparta, MI 49345
Phone: (616) 453-1477
www.paactusa.org

Prostate Cancer Foundation
1250 Fourth Street
Santa Monica, CA 90401
Phone: (800) 757-2873
www.pcf.org

The Prostate Net, Inc.
P.O. Box 10188
Newark, NJ 07101
Phone: (201) 289-8221
www.prostatenet.org

Us Too!
2720 South River Road, Suite 112
Des Plains, IL 60018
Phone: (630) 795-1002
Toll free: (800) 808-7866
www.ustoo.org

ZERO—The Project to End Prostate Cancer
515 King Street, Suite 420
Alexandria, VA 22314
Phone: (202) 463-9455
www.zerocancer.org

Glossary

acute bacterial prostatitis: a sudden severe prostate infection caused by bacteria.

adjuvant therapy: a treatment added to the primary treatment.

adrenal glands: a pair of small glands, one on top of each kidney, that produce small amounts of the male hormone testosterone.

agonist: a drug that simulates physiologic activity at cell receptors stimulated by naturally occurring substances.

alpha-adrenergic agonists: vasoconstrictors (substances that constrict the blood vessels); decongestants.

anastomosis: surgical reattachment of the urethra to the bladder neck after prostatectomy.

androgen blockade: therapy used to eliminate male sex hormones in the body.

androgen deprivation: a treatment that prevents male hormones, principally testosterone, from feeding prostate cancer cells.

androgen-independent cancer: a prostate malignancy that does not depend on male hormones to grow and divide.

androgens: male hormones, including testosterone.

anemia: low red blood cell count.

angiogenesis: the growth of blood vessels.

antagonist: in medicine, a substance that blocks the action of a drug, hormone, or cell.

antiandrogen: a substance that saturates androgen receptors in the prostate and blocks access of testosterone and DHT to those receptors.

antibody: substances the body produces to defend against disease.

anticholinergic agents: drugs that block the neurotransmitter acetylcholine. May be used for urinary urgency.

antioxidants: chemicals (including nutrients such as vitamins A, C, and E) that reduce or prevent oxidation, especially within tissues.

apoptosis: the normal cell death and replacement process.

atypia: variation (indicating disease) in the appearance of the centers of body cells as viewed under a microscope. *See also* prostatic intraepithelial neuroplasia (PIN).

autologous donation: giving your own blood to be used if you need a transfusion during or after surgery.

B

B-mode acquisition and targeting (BAT): an ultrasound positioning system used in the radiation treatment of prostate cancer to localize targets that may move from one treatment day to the next.

benign: in medicine, noncancerous.

benign prostatic hyperplasia (BPH): prostate enlargement caused by growth of tissue surrounding the urethra.

beta carotene: a nutrient related to vitamin A that is found in dark green and dark yellow fruits and vegetables.

biomarkers: naturally occurring body substances whose fluctuations sometimes indicate cancer.

biopsy: removal of a sample of body tissue for pathological examination.

bisphosphonates: a class of drugs used to prevent or treat osteoporosis.

bone marrow: the soft, spongy centers of large bones where blood cells are made.

bone scan: an imaging study that creates images of bones on a computer screen for diagnosis.

brachytherapy: a procedure in which radioactive seeds are implanted in the body to kill cancer cells.

C

cancer: disease characterized by uncontrolled growth and spread of abnormal cells.

castration level: little or no measurable PSA, as would be achieved by surgical castration.

CAT/CT scan: computerized axial tomography. *See* computerized tomography scan.

central zone: refers to the prostate gland's muscular central zone, which prevents semen from backing up into the bladder during ejaculation.

chemical castration: the use of drugs to reduce testosterone to the level that would be achieved with orchiectomy.

chemotherapy: treatment with anti-cancer drugs.

chronic bacterial prostatitis: persistent and recurrent inflammation of the prostate caused by bacteria.

Cialis: a PDE-5 inhibitor used to treat impotence and erectile dysfunction; generic, tadalafil.

clinical stage: the suspected extent of cancer's spread using evidence gathered from pretreatment testing. See also pathologic stage; stage.

colony stimulating factors: drugs that promote white blood cell production.

colostomy: a surgical procedure in which the large intestine is routed to an opening in the body through which fecal waste passes to an external bag.

computerized tomography scan (CT or CAT scan): a diagnostic method that uses computerized X-ray images to create a three-dimensional picture of an internal part of the body.

conformal EBRT: a type of external beam radiation therapy in which the radiation beams are more precisely targeted at a patient's tumor than is the case in conventional EBRT.

continence: in medicine, voluntary control over urination and defecation.

corpora cavernosa: the two parallel chambers of the penis that fill with blood to produce an erection.

corpus spongiosum: a central chamber in the penis through which the urethra passes.

cryoablation: destruction of diseased or damaged tissue by freezing.

cryolumpectomy: a procedure in which supercooled cryoprobes are used to destroy a tumor and a minimal amount of surrounding tissue rather than the entire gland in which the tumor resides.

cryoprobes: supercooled instruments used in cryotherapy.

cryosurgery: see cryoablation.

cryotherapy: a medical treatment that destroys abnormal tissues by freezing.

CT/CAT scan: *see* computerized tomography scan.

D

debulking: in oncology, reducing the size of a tumor with one treatment, such as hormone therapy or chemotherapy, to facilitate another treatment, such as radiation, cryoablation, or surgery.

deep venous thrombosis: blood clots in the deep veins of the legs.

DEH: *see* diethylstilbestrol.

Denonvillier's fascia: a thin sheet of tissue that separates the prostate and the rectum.

DHT: *see* dihydrotestosterone.

diethylstilbestrol (DES): a form of estrogen.

differentiated: in pathology, a term applied to cells with distinct borders and centers.

diffuse: widespread, scattered, or dispersed.

digital rectal examination (DRE): a diagnostic procedure in which a doctor inserts a gloved, lubricated finger into a man's rectum and feels through the back rectal wall for abnormalities.

dihydrotestosterone (DHT): a potent male hormone to which testosterone is converted in the prostate.

DRE: *see* digital rectal examination.

DVT: *see* deep venous thrombosis

E

EBRT: *see* external beam radiation therapy.

ejaculatory duct: a channel leading from the seminal vesicle and the vas deferens through the prostate that carries semen out of the body at the time of ejaculation.

endoscope: a long, slender medical instrument equipped with a small camera for examining the interior of an organ or performing surgery.

epididymis: a thin, tightly coiled tube that carries sperm from the testicle to the vas deferens.

epidural: the space between the wall of the spinal canal and the covering of the spinal cord; an anesthetic injection or infusion into this space.

estrogen: a sex hormone that regulates women's reproduction, sometimes used as hormone therapy to treat prostate cancer in men.

external beam radiation therapy (EBRT; XRT): a procedure that uses radiation to destroy cancer from outside the body.

extravasation injury: damage that occurs around the injection site when chemotherapy drugs leak into nearby tissues.

F

Foley catheter: an indwelling catheter—a tube usually inserted for the removal of body waste—that remains in the urethra and bladder until removed.

follicle-stimulating hormone (FSH): a substance that stimulates the testicles to produce testosterone.

free PSA: protein specific antigens that circulate in the blood and are not attached to protein molecules.

free radicals: oxidants; unstable high-energy particles in the body that damage cells.

G

Gleason score: a number between 2 and 10 in a system of grading prostate cancer cells. The lower the number, the closer to normal the cells appear. In general, the higher the number, the more aggressive the tumor.

grade: in oncology, a measure of tumor cells' abnormality and aggressiveness.

granulocytopenia: low white blood cell count.

gynecomastia: breast enlargement and tenderness in men.

H

hematospermia: blood in the semen.

hematuria: blood in the urine.

high-dose-rate implantation (HDR): a brachytherapy procedure in which very high-energy radioactive wires are implanted, left in the body for a short time, then removed.

hormone therapy: in prostate cancer, a treatment whose purpose is to block the body's production, circulation, or absorption of testosterone.

hyperplasia: a benign growth, a thickening or overgrowth of cells.

I

immobilization device: a form-fitting apparatus that helps patients lie perfectly still during external beam radiation therapy.

impotence: the inability to have an erection.

IMRT: *see* intensity-modulated radiation therapy.

incontinence: *see* urinary incontinence.

infusion: in medicine, a method of introducing ("dripping") fluids, including drugs, into the bloodstream.

intensity-modulated radiation therapy (IMRT): in external beam radiation therapy, a technique using multiple small beams that come together to form a single conformal radiation beam.

K

Kegel exercises: a type of muscle training that involves systematically tightening and releasing the urinary sphincter to control the flow of urine.

L

laparoscope: an endoscope (a thin, camera-equipped medical instrument) inserted through a small incision in the abdomen for examination or surgery.

laparoscopic pelvic lymphadenectomy: removal of lymph nodes, using a laparoscope, for pathological examination.

Levitra: a PDE-5 inhibitor used to treat erectile dysfunction or impotence; generic, vardenafil.

LHRH: *see* luteinizing hormone releasing hormone.

LHRH agonist: a substance that tells the pituitary gland to stop producing LHRH.

linear accelerator: a high-energy X-ray treatment machine.

lumpectomy: surgical removal of a tumor and a minimal amount of surrounding tissue rather than the entire gland in which the tumor resides.

luteinizing hormone (LH): a substance that stimulates the testicles to produce testosterone.

luteinizing hormone releasing hormone (LHRH): a substance that stimulates the pituitary gland to release luteinizing hormone.

lycopene: a red pigment (a form of carotenoid) that gives tomatoes their red color and that may help prevent prostate cancer.

lymph: thin clear fluid containing white blood cells that travels through the body's lymphatic system and helps fight infection and disease.

lymphadenectomy: a procedure in which lymph nodes are removed from the body to be examined for cancer.

M

magnetic resonance imaging (MRI): a noninvasive procedure that creates a two-dimensional picture of an internal organ or structure. Magnetic resonance imaging, unlike computerized tomography and X-rays, for example, does not involve radiation.

malignant: in medicine, cancerous.

medical castration: *see* chemical castration.

medical oncologist: A doctor who has special training in diagnosing and treating cancer in adults using chemotherapy, hormonal therapy, biological therapy, and targeted therapy.

metastases: cancerous tumors that spread from the original site.

metastasize: spread, as cancer cells.

minilap: *see* minilaparotomy staging pelvic lymphadenectomy.

minilaparotomy staging pelvic lymphadenectomy: a surgical procedure that takes place immediately before radical prostatectomy. A surgeon removes pelvic lymph nodes through a small incision. If they are found to contain cancer, the prostatectomy is generally canceled.

MRI: *see* magnetic resonance imaging.

multifocal prostate cancer: malignant tumors at several sites within the prostate.

N

nanogram: one-billionth of a gram.

needle biopsy: removal of suspected cancer cells through a hollow needle (rather than during a surgical procedure).

neoadjuvant therapy: a treatment given before the primary treatment.

nerve-sparing prostatectomy: surgical removal of the prostate gland that leaves one or both nearby neurovascular bundles intact.

neuropathy: nerve damage expressed as tingling or loss of sensation in the hands or feet.

neurovascular bundles: clusters of nerves near the prostate that enable men to have erections.

neutropenia: low white blood cell count.

nonbacterial prostatitis: inflammation of the prostate from an unknown cause.

O

orchiectomy: surgical castration (removal of the testicles).

organ-confined: of cancer, a tumor or tumors that have not breached the original site.

osteoporosis: a condition of decreased bone mass. This leads to fragile bones which are at an increased risk for fractures.

overflow incontinence: urine leakage that occurs when normal urine flow is blocked and the bladder is always full.

oxidants: *see* free radicals.

P

palliative: used to relieve symptoms rather than cure the underlying illness.

Partin Tables: a tool that uses PSA, clinical stage, and Gleason score to predict how a prostate cancer is likely to behave.

pathologic stage: the actual extent to which a cancer has spread as determined by pathological examination of tissue removed during surgery. *See also* clinical stage; stage.

pathologist: a medical doctor who specializes in examining tissue to make a diagnosis.

patient-controlled analgesia (PCA pump): a pump system for self-administering pain medication. Though patients control their own dosages, the system has safeguards against dosing too much or too often.

PCA pump: *see* patient-controlled analgesia.

PDE-5 inhibitors: drugs used to treat erectile dysfunction and impotence.

pelvic-floor exercises: *see* Kegel exercises.

percutaneous: through unbroken skin.

perineum: the area between the anus and the scrotum.

peripheral zone: the largest part of the prostate, containing about three-fourths of the glands in the prostate.

permanent seed implant (PSI): the permanent implantation of radioactive seeds in the prostate gland.

PET scan: *see* positron-emission tomography scan.

phytoestrogens: naturally occurring estrogen-like compounds found in plants.

PIN: *see* prostatic intraepithelial neoplasia.

pituitary gland: located at the base of the brain, the master gland of the endocrine system.

planning study: preparations made for the delivery of radiation therapy.

pneumatic stockings: devices worn on the legs during and after surgery to improve circulation by repeatedly inflating and deflating.

positive margin: cancer identified at the cut surface (incision) of the prostate after surgical removal.

positron-emission tomography (PET) scan: a computerized image of body tissues' metabolic activity to determine the presence of disease.

ProstaScint: a staging tool similar to a bone scan except that it finds "hot spots" in soft tissue rather than bones.

prostate capsule: the membrane that encases the numerous small glands of the prostate.

prostate gland: a firm, partly muscular, walnut-sized gland in males at the base of the bladder; produces a secretion that is the fluid part of semen.

prostate-specific antigen (PSA): a protein manufactured by the prostate to help liquefy semen. Elevated PSA levels can signal prostate disease.

prostatic intraepithelial neoplasia (PIN): cell abnormalities sometimes described as precancerous. *See also* atypia.

prostatitis: inflammation of the prostate.

PSA: *see* prostate-specific antigen.

PSA velocity: the rate at which PSA levels rise.

pubis: one of the pelvic bones.

pulmonary embolism: a blood clot in the lung.

R

radiation oncologist: a medical doctor who specializes in using radiation to treat cancer.

radical laparoscopic prostatectomy: surgical removal of the prostate through a small abdominal incision using an endoscope.

radical perineal prostatectomy: a surgical procedure in which the prostate is removed through an incision in the perineum.

radical prostatectomy: a surgical procedure in which the prostate, seminal vesicles, and pelvic lymph nodes are removed through an incision in the lower abdomen.

radioactive seeds: energy-emitting pellets implanted to kill cancer cells.

radioresistant: of tumors, those that are not easily destroyed by radiation therapy.

S

salvage therapy: in prostate cancer, a follow-up treatment used when the primary treatment has failed to eradicate the disease.

saturation biopsy: a biopsy in which specimens are obtained at 5-mm intervals throughout the prostate. Carried out through the perineum under ultrasound guidance.

seed implantation: a procedure in which radioactive seeds are placed in the body to kill cancer cells.

semen: a milky liquid produced by the seminal vesicles to carry sperm out of the body.

seminal fluid: fluid from the prostate and other sex glands that helps transport sperm during orgasm.

seminal vesicles: small organs alongside the prostate that manufacture semen.

sepsis: a serious illness caused by severe infection of the bloodstream by a toxin-producing bacteria, virus, or fungus.

stage: of cancer, the extent to which a tumor has spread from its primary site. *See also* clinical stage; pathologic stage.

staging pelvic lymphadenectomy: removal of pelvic lymph nodes to determine whether cancer has spread from the prostate.

stress urinary incontinence: involuntary leakage of urine caused by activity or the sudden movement involved in sneezing, coughing, or laughing.

surgical castration: *see* orchiectomy.

T

three-dimensional map biopsy: *see* saturation biopsy.

temporary seed implant: *see* high-dose-rate implantation (HDR).

testes: *see* testicles.

testicles: the principal organs where the male hormone testosterone is produced.

testosterone: the predominant male hormone, responsible for most male-related traits.

thrombocytopenia: low blood platelet level.

TNM staging system: method of classifying malignant tumors with respect to primary tumor, involvement of regional lymph nodes, and presence or absence of metastastes.

transrectal ultrasound (TRUS): an imaging technique in which sound waves produce a "picture" of the prostate and abnormalities it might contain.

transurethral resection of the prostate (TURP): surgery to remove prostate tissue through the urethra to treat benign prostatic hyperplasia.

TRUS: *see* transrectal ultrasound.

tumor: a mass of abnormal cells, which may be malignant (cancerous) or benign (noncancerous).

tumor markers: *see* biomarkers.

TURP: *see* transurethral resection of the prostate.

U

unifocal prostate cancer: a single malignant tumor within the prostate.

ureters: tubes that carry urine from the kidneys to the bladder.

urethra: the duct through which urine leaves the body; also, in males, the genital duct.

urethral stricture: narrowing of the urethra caused by scar tissue that forms after surgery.

urethrorectal fistula: a hole between the digestive and urinary tracts.

urge incontinence: the inability to hold urine long enough to reach a restroom.

urinary bladder: the organ in which urine is stored after leaving the kidneys and before leaving the body.

urinary incontinence: inability to control the leaking of urine from the body.

urinary sphincter: the ring of muscle that contracts to prevent urine from leaking.

urologist: a physician who has special knowledge of the male and female urinary tract and the male reproductive organs.

V

vas deferens: singular form of vasa deferentia.

vasa deferentia: the tubes that carry sperm out of the testicles.

vasodilator: a drug that widens blood vessels.

venous access device: a port, under the skin, usually in the chest area, for accessing veins to administer medications intravenously.

Viagra: a PDE-5 inhibitor used to treat erectile dysfunction or impotence; generic, sildenafil citrate.

W

Whitmore-Jewett staging system: a method of describing prostate cancer's spread, less commonly used than the TNM staging system.

X

XRT: *see* external beam radiation therapy

Index

Index

About the Author

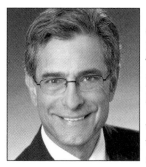

Arthur S. Centeno, M.D., is a board-certified urologist in private practice at Urology San Antonio in San Antonio, Texas. He has treated prostate cancer patients through surgery, brachytherapy, and cryosurgery.

"I decided I wanted to be a doctor when I was twelve years old and while visiting my grandfather in the hospital and I realized I wanted to help people. My philosophy of medicine has evolved over the years. I have learned it is important that doctors be more than medical technologists—they must also be empathetic to patients and families. This became so clear to me when my wife died of breast cancer in 2001. I teach my medical students that we are dealing with people, not just diseases."

Dr. Centeno is a graduate of the University of Texas Health Science Center in San Antonio, Texas. He completed his surgical internship and residency in urology at the University of Texas Medical Branch in Galveston, Texas, and earned a Master of Medical Sciences degree at that institution's Graduate School of Biomedical Sciences.

Dr. Centeno has served as president of the Texas Urological Society; he is a member of the American Urological Association and Sigma Xi Scientific Research Society. He is a Fellow of the American College of Surgeons. He has two children, Rebecca and Everett.

Dr. Centeno may be reached at:
www.urologysanantonio.com.

117

Consumer Health Titles from Addicus Books

Visit our online catalog at www.AddicusBooks.com

To Order Books:
Visit us online at: www.AddicusBooks.com
Call toll free: (800) 888-4741

For discounts on bulk purchases, call our Special Sales
Department at (402) 330-7493.
Or email us at: info@Addicus Books.com

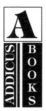

Addicus Books
P. O. Box 45327
Omaha, NE 68145

*Addicus Books is dedicated to publishing consumer health books
that comfort and educate.*